GULF WAR and HEALTH

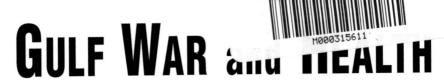

Treatment for
Chronic Multisymptom Illness

Committee on Gulf War and Health:
Treatment for Chronic Multisymptom Illness

Board on the Health of Select Populations

INSTITUTE OF MEDICINE
OF THE NATIONAL ACADEMIES

THE NATIONAL ACADEMIES PRESS
Washington, D.C.
www.nap.edu

THE NATIONAL ACADEMIES PRESS   500 Fifth Street, NW   Washington, DC 20001

NOTICE: The project that is the subject of this report was approved by the Governing Board of the National Research Council, whose members are drawn from the councils of the National Academy of Sciences, the National Academy of Engineering, and the Institute of Medicine. The members of the committee responsible for the report were chosen for their special competences and with regard for appropriate balance.

This study was supported by Contract VA241-P-2024 between the National Academy of Sciences and the Department of Veterans Affairs. Any opinions, findings, conclusions, or recommendations expressed in this publication are those of the authors and do not necessarily reflect the views of the organizations or agencies that provided support for the project.

International Standard Book Number-13:   978-0-309-27802-7
International Standard Book Number-10:   0-309-27802-3

Additional copies of this report are available for sale from the National Academies Press, 500 Fifth Street, NW, Keck 360, Washington, DC 20001; (800) 624-6242 or (202) 334-3313; Internet, http://www.nap.edu.

For more information about the Institute of Medicine, visit the IOM home page at: www.iom.edu.

The serpent has been a symbol of long life, healing, and knowledge among almost all cultures and religions since the beginning of recorded history. The serpent adopted as a logotype by the Institute of Medicine is a relief carving from ancient Greece, now held by the Staatliche Museen in Berlin.

Suggested citation: IOM (Institute of Medicine). 2013. *Gulf War and Health: Treatment for Chronic Multisymptom Illness*. Washington, DC: The National Academies Press.

*"Knowing is not enough; we must apply.
Willing is not enough; we must do."*
—Goethe

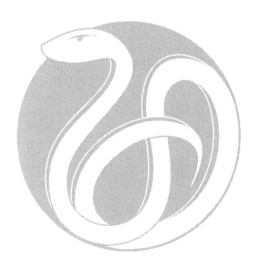

INSTITUTE OF MEDICINE
OF THE NATIONAL ACADEMIES

Advising the Nation. Improving Health.

THE NATIONAL ACADEMIES
Advisers to the Nation on Science, Engineering, and Medicine

The **National Academy of Sciences** is a private, nonprofit, self-perpetuating society of distinguished scholars engaged in scientific and engineering research, dedicated to the furtherance of science and technology and to their use for the general welfare. Upon the authority of the charter granted to it by the Congress in 1863, the Academy has a mandate that requires it to advise the federal government on scientific and technical matters. Dr. Ralph J. Cicerone is president of the National Academy of Sciences.

The **National Academy of Engineering** was established in 1964, under the charter of the National Academy of Sciences, as a parallel organization of outstanding engineers. It is autonomous in its administration and in the selection of its members, sharing with the National Academy of Sciences the responsibility for advising the federal government. The National Academy of Engineering also sponsors engineering programs aimed at meeting national needs, encourages education and research, and recognizes the superior achievements of engineers. Dr. Charles M. Vest is president of the National Academy of Engineering.

The **Institute of Medicine** was established in 1970 by the National Academy of Sciences to secure the services of eminent members of appropriate professions in the examination of policy matters pertaining to the health of the public. The Institute acts under the responsibility given to the National Academy of Sciences by its congressional charter to be an adviser to the federal government and, upon its own initiative, to identify issues of medical care, research, and education. Dr. Harvey V. Fineberg is president of the Institute of Medicine.

The **National Research Council** was organized by the National Academy of Sciences in 1916 to associate the broad community of science and technology with the Academy's purposes of furthering knowledge and advising the federal government. Functioning in accordance with general policies determined by the Academy, the Council has become the principal operating agency of both the National Academy of Sciences and the National Academy of Engineering in providing services to the government, the public, and the scientific and engineering communities. The Council is administered jointly by both Academies and the Institute of Medicine. Dr. Ralph J. Cicerone and Dr. Charles M. Vest are chair and vice chair, respectively, of the National Research Council.

www.national-academies.org

Staff

ABIGAIL MITCHELL, Study Director
CARY HAVER, Associate Program Officer
JONATHAN SCHMELZER, Senior Program Assistant
NORMAN GROSSBLATT, Senior Editor
GARY WALKER, Financial Officer
JIM BANIHASHEMI, Financial Officer
FREDERICK ERDTMANN, Director, Board on the Health of Select
    Populations

Reviewers

This report has been reviewed in draft form by persons chosen for their diverse perspectives and technical expertise in accordance with procedures approved by the National Research Council's Report Review Committee. The purpose of this independent review is to provide candid and critical comments that will assist the institution in making its published report as sound as possible and to ensure that the report meets institutional standards of objectivity, evidence, and responsiveness to the study charge. The review comments and draft manuscript remain confidential to protect the integrity of the deliberative process. We thank the following for their review of the report:

Niloofar Afari, University of California, San Diego
Melvin S. Blanchard, Washington University School of Medicine
Paul W. Brandt-Rauf, University of Illinois at Chicago School of Public Health
Sandro Galea, Columbia University Mailman School of Public Health
Naomi L. Gerber, George Mason University
Thomas V. Holohan, Clinical Evaluation, LLC; formerly Veterans Health Administration
David R. Nerenz, Henry Ford Health System
Eliseo J. Perez-Stable, University of California, San Francisco
Karen S. Quigley, Northeastern University and Edith Nourse Rogers Memorial VA Medical Center
Sandra J. W. Smeeding, Veterans Affairs Salt Lake City Health Care System
Nancy Fugate Woods, University of Washington School of Nursing

Although the reviewers listed above have provided many constructive comments and suggestions, they were not asked to endorse the conclusions or recommendations, nor did they see the final draft of the report before its release. The review of the report was overseen by **Lynn R. Goldman,** Dean, the George Washington University School of Public Health and Health Services, and **Enriqueta C. Bond,** President Emeritus, Burroughs Wellcome Fund. Appointed by the National Research Council and the Institute of Medicine, respectively, they were responsible for making certain that an independent examination of the report was carried out in accordance with institutional procedures and that all review comments were carefully considered. Responsibility for the final content of the report rests entirely with the authoring committee and the institution.

Preface

The committee was convened to review, evaluate, and summarize the available scientific and medical literature regarding the best treatments for chronic multisymptom illness (CMI) in Gulf War veterans. We accepted that responsibility in recognition of the personal and family sacrifices that all soldiers—both deployed and nondeployed—undertake in times of conflict. About 700,000 military personnel served in the 1991 Gulf War, and as of September 2011, about 2.6 million military personnel had been deployed to the Iraq and Afghanistan wars. There is no script for the stresses that are endured; they are personal and many. The committee was most appreciative of the willingness of many veterans to share their experiences and thoughts with us so that we would be better prepared to move forward with our task. We undertook a thorough review of the studies[1] already completed by the Institute of Medicine (IOM) on this general topic and then expanded the evidence base by conducting a systematic search of the available scientific and medical literature regarding the best treatments for CMI. The committee evaluated the evidence by using the scientifically rigorous process detailed in this report. As we approached the task at hand, we stood firm on the concerns for patient-centered care and our abilities to communicate our thoughts, conclusions, and recommendations to all interested audiences.

---

[1]IOM (Institute of Medicine). 2001. *Gulf War Veterans: Treating Symptoms and Syndromes.* Washington, DC: National Academy Press; IOM. 2010. *Gulf War and Health, Volume 8: Update of Health Effects of Serving in the Gulf War.* Washington, DC: The National Academies Press.

To focus our efforts, we defined CMI as the presence of a spectrum of chronic symptoms experienced for 6 months or longer in at least two of six categories—fatigue, mood and cognition, musculoskeletal, gastrointestinal, respiratory, and neurologic—that may overlap with but are not fully captured by known syndromes (such as irritable bowel syndrome, chronic fatigue syndrome, and fibromyalgia) or other diagnoses.

Our review of the literature revealed that specific etiologic agents or histopathologic findings often are not associated with such symptoms, and the causes of many of the symptoms ascribed to CMI remain unknown. However, the lack of diagnostic and etiologic clarity does not undermine the legitimacy of the reports of the symptoms. The multiple manifestations of the symptoms make directed treatment more challenging, and clinicians are often frustrated by the difficulties in managing care for people who have CMI. However, for veterans whose function and life satisfaction are limited by their symptoms, it remains no less important.

We hope that our recommendations will make a difference in the lives of people who have CMI. It is clear that this condition has adversely affected the health and well-being of a substantial number of our veterans and their families. Anecdotal reports appear regularly in the mass media.[2] We encourage the Department of Veterans Affairs (VA) to apply the principles set forth in this report, including at a minimum adequate resources to ensure early entry into the VA health care system and adherence to the principles of patient-centered and compassionate care, shared decision making, and regular clinical follow-up as necessary. Our veterans deserve the very best health care.

The committee thanks everyone who presented and participated in discussions during the public meetings, which informed our work and helped us to develop our approach to and thought process regarding the statement of task. The wide variety of viewpoints were expressed during those information sessions provided valuable insight into the complexity of medical treatment for CMI in Gulf War veterans. The time and effort to travel to the public meetings and prepare written materials and statements are greatly appreciated.

The committee is particularly appreciative of the many Gulf War veterans who spoke and submitted written accounts of their experiences in the gulf and on their return to the United States. They provided valuable understanding of the symptoms and medical conditions of CMI and of medical treatment for it as experienced by the many men and women who served in the Gulf War.

The committee also owes a debt of gratitude to the following persons who traveled to and presented valuable information at our public meetings:

---

[2]For example, Kristof, N. D. 2012. War wounds. *New York Times*, August 10, SR1.

Caroline Blaum, University of Michigan Health System; Daniel Clauw, University of Michigan Health System; Jeffery Dusek, Abbott Northwestern Hospital; Charles Engel, Deployment Health Clinical Center; Beatrice Golomb, University of California, San Diego, School of Medicine and San Diego VA Medical Center; Stephen Hunt, VA Puget Sound Health Care System; Kenneth Kendler, Virginia Commonwealth University; Kurt Kroenke, Regenstrief Institute; Ronald Poropatich, US Army Medical Research and Materiel Command; and Matt Reinhard, War-Related Illness and Injury Study Center, Washington, DC.

The committee thanks Patrick Furey of Consumersphere, a consultant who provided an analysis of the social media discussion surrounding CMI in veterans of the Gulf War. We also thank Michael Peterson and Terry Walters, of the VA Office of Public Health, for providing helpful background information.

I would like to thank the committee members for their time commitment to this important project, their diligence in reviewing every detail of complex issues, and their sensitivity to the concerns of our veterans. Finally, I thank the IOM staff for their thoroughness, knowledge, research expertise, and guidance throughout this journey to try to make a contribution to the understanding of a complex subject.

Bernard M. Rosof, *Chair*
Committee on Gulf War and Health:
Treatment for Chronic Multisymptom Illness

Contents

Boxes, Figures, and Tables

BOXES

FIGURES

TABLES

Abbreviations and Acronyms

AACH American Academy on Communication in Healthcare
ACP American College of Physicians
AHRQ Agency for Healthcare Research and Quality
ALS amyotrophic lateral sclerosis
AMSTAR Assessment of Multiple Systematic Reviews
AOC alteration of consciousness
APA American Psychiatric Association

BMI body mass index

CACTUS Classical Acupuncture Treatment for People with
Unexplained Symptoms
CAM complementary and alternative medicine
CBOC community-based outpatient clinic
CBT cognitive behavioral therapy
CDC Centers for Disease Control and Prevention
CFS chronic fatigue syndrome
CI confidence interval
CINAHL Cumulative Index to Nursing and Allied Health Literature
CMI chronic multisymptom illness
CPAP continuous positive airway pressure
CPG clinical practice guideline
CQI continuous quality improvement
CRT cognitive rehabilitation therapy

DARE   Database of Abstracts of Reviews of Effects
DNA   deoxyribonucleic acid
DOD   Department of Defense
DSM   *Diagnostic and Statistical Manual of Mental Disorders*
DU   depleted uranium

EBI   evidence-based information
ECHO   Extension for Community Healthcare Outcomes
ECT   electroconvulsive therapy
EMC   enhanced medical care
EMDR   eye-movement desensitization and reprocessing

FD   functional dyspepsia
FDA   Food and Drug Administration
FGID   functional gastrointestinal disorder
FPOW   former prisoner of war
FSS   functional somatic syndrome
FY   fiscal year

GET   graded exercise therapy
GI   gastrointestinal
GMT   geographically adjusted income threshold
GWI   Gulf War illness
GWV   Gulf War–deployed veterans
GWVI   Gulf War veterans illness

IBS   irritable bowel syndrome
ICT   information and communication technology
IHI   Institute for Health Improvement
IOM   Institute of Medicine

LOC   loss of consciousness

ME   myalgic encephalomyelitis
MI   motivational interviewing
mTBI   mild traumatic brain injury
MUPS   medically unexplained physical symptoms
MUS   medically unexplained symptoms

NHS   National Health Service (UK)
NICE   National Institute for Health and Clinical Excellence (UK)
NSAID   nonsteroidal anti-inflammatory drug

OEF	Operation Enduring Freedom
OIF	Operation Iraqi Freedom
OND	Operation New Dawn
OR	odds ratio
PC	primary care
PCMH	patient-centered medical home
PCS	postconcussive symptom
PD-PACT	postdeployment patient-aligned care team
PIT	psychodynamic interpersonal therapy
PTA	posttraumatic amnesia
PTSD	posttraumatic stress disorder
RAC	VA Research Advisory Committee on Gulf War Veterans' Illnesses
RCT	randomized controlled trial
REAC-BS	radioelectric asymmetric brain stimulation
REM	rapid eye movement
RoB	risk of bias
SCAN	Specialty Care Access Network
SHAD	Shipboard Hazard and Defense
SIGLE	System for Information on Grey Literature in Europe
SNRI	serotonin norepinephrine reuptake inhibitor
SSD	somatic symptom disorder
SSRI	selective serotonin reuptake inhibitor
TBI	traumatic brain injury
TENS	transcutaneous electric nerve stimulation
UK	United Kingdom
VA	Department of Veterans Affairs
VAMC	VA medical center
VA-OIG	VA Office of the Inspector General
VBA	Veterans Benefits Administration
VHA	Veterans Health Administration
VISN	Veterans Integrated Service Network
WGO	World Gastroenterology Organisation
WRIISC	War-Related Illness and Injury Study Center

Summary

Chronic multisymptom illness (CMI) is a serious condition that imposes an enormous burden of suffering on our nation's veterans. Veterans who have CMI often have physical symptoms (such as fatigue, joint and muscle pain, and gastrointestinal symptoms) and cognitive symptoms (such as memory difficulties) and may have comorbid syndromes with shared symptoms (such as chronic fatigue syndrome [CFS], fibromyalgia, and irritable bowel syndrome [IBS]) and other clinical entities (such as depression and anxiety). For the purposes of this report, the committee defined CMI as the presence of a spectrum of chronic symptoms experienced for 6 months or longer in at least two of six categories—fatigue, mood and cognition, musculoskeletal, gastrointestinal, respiratory, and neurologic—that may overlap with but are not fully captured by known syndromes (such as CFS, fibromyalgia, and IBS) or other diagnoses.

Despite considerable efforts by researchers in the United States and elsewhere, there is no consensus among physicians, researchers, and others as to the cause of CMI. There is a growing belief that no specific causal factor or agent will be identified.

Many thousands of Gulf War veterans[1] who have CMI live with sometimes debilitating symptoms and seek an effective way to manage their symp-

_____

[1]Veterans are considered to have served in the Gulf War if they were on active military duty in the Southwest Asia theater of military operations during the period from the 1991 Gulf War (Operation Desert Storm) through the Iraq War (Operation Iraqi Freedom and Operation New Dawn). Although Afghanistan is not in the Southwest Asia theater of operations, for the purpose of this report veterans of the Afghanistan War (Operation Enduring Freedom) are included in the Gulf War veteran population.

1

toms. Estimates of the numbers of 1991 Gulf War veterans who have CMI range from 175,000 to 250,000 (about 25–35% of the 1991 Gulf War veteran population), and there is evidence that CMI in 1991 Gulf War veterans may not resolve over time. Preliminary data suggest that CMI is occurring in veterans of the Iraq and Afghanistan wars as well. In 2010, a previous committee of the Institute of Medicine (IOM) recommended "a renewed research effort with substantial commitment to well-organized efforts to better identify and treat multisymptom illness in Gulf War veterans" (IOM, 2010).

THE CHARGE TO THE COMMITTEE

The present study was mandated by Congress in the Veterans Benefits Act of 2010 (Public Law 111-275, October 13, 2010). That law directs the secretary of veterans affairs "to enter into an agreement with the Institute of Medicine of the National Academies to carry out a comprehensive review of the best treatments for CMI in Persian Gulf War veterans and an evaluation of how such treatment approaches could best be disseminated throughout the Department of Veterans Affairs [VA] to improve the care and benefits provided to veterans." In August 2011, VA asked that IOM conduct a study to address that charge, and IOM appointed the Committee on Gulf War and Health: Treatment for Chronic Multisymptom Illness. The complete charge to the committee follows.

> The IOM will convene a committee to comprehensively review, evaluate, and summarize the available scientific and medical literature regarding the best treatments for chronic multisymptom illness among Gulf War veterans.
>
> In its evaluation, the committee will look broadly for relevant information. Information sources to pursue could include, but are not limited to:
>
> - Published peer-reviewed literature concerning the treatment of multisymptom illness among the 1991 Gulf War veteran population;
> - Published peer-reviewed literature concerning treatment of multisymptom illness among Operation Enduring Freedom, Operation Iraqi Freedom, and Operation New Dawn active-duty service members and veterans;
> - Published peer-reviewed literature concerning treatment of multisymptom illness among similar populations such as allied military personnel; and
> - Published peer-reviewed literature concerning treatment of populations with a similar constellation of symptoms.
>
> In addition to summarizing the available scientific and medical literature regarding the best treatments for chronic multisymptom illness among Gulf War veterans, the IOM will:

- Recommend how best to disseminate this information throughout the VA to improve the care and benefits provided to veterans.
- Recommend additional scientific studies and research initiatives to resolve areas of continuing scientific uncertainty.
- Recommend such legislative or administrative action as the IOM deems appropriate in light of the results of its review.

THE COMMITTEE'S APPROACH TO ITS CHARGE

A multipronged approach was used to respond to the charge. A systematic review was conducted to evaluate the scientific literature on therapies to eliminate or alleviate the symptoms associated with, or that define, CMI. Because many people who have CMI also have other unexplained conditions with shared symptoms (such as CFS, fibromyalgia, and IBS) and may have comorbid conditions (such as depression and anxiety), treatments recommended in guidelines or supported by evidence as summarized in systematic reviews for these related and comorbid conditions also were reviewed to identify any treatments potentially beneficial in people who have CMI.

Managing patients who have CMI involves more than administering a therapy. It requires a broader view of treatment. To explore other aspects of care, the committee drew on multiple sources (such as the scientific literature, government reports, care programs used by organizations, an analysis of social media, and testimony from veterans and their families) so that it could make recommendations to VA about improving its model of care for veterans who have CMI, educating VA clinicians to improve their knowledge about how to care for these patients, and improving communication between clinicians and patients who have CMI.

FINDINGS, CONCLUSIONS, AND RECOMMENDATIONS

The committee's findings, conclusions, and recommendations are in five major categories:

1. Treatments for CMI.
2. The VA health care system as it is related to improving systems of care and the management of care for veterans who have CMI.
3. Dissemination of information through the VA health care system about caring for veterans who have CMI.
4. Improving the collection and quality of data on outcomes and satisfaction of care for veterans who have CMI and are treated in VA health care facilities.
5. Research on diagnosing and treating CMI and on program evaluation.

Treatments for Chronic Multisymptom Illness

The committee conducted a de novo systematic assessment of the evidence on treatments for symptoms associated with CMI. The committee also identified evidence-based guidelines and systematic reviews on treatments for related and comorbid conditions (fibromyalgia, chronic pain, CFS, somatic symptom disorders, sleep disorders, IBS, functional dyspepsia, depression, anxiety, posttraumatic stress disorder, traumatic brain injury, substance-use and addictive disorders, and self-harm) to determine whether any treatments found to be effective for one of these conditions may be beneficial for CMI. Both pharmacologic and nonpharmacologic treatments were assessed. Holistic and integrative treatment approaches were considered in addition to individual interventions.

Studies of treatments for the symptoms associated with CMI conducted in the 1991 Gulf War veteran population were included in the assessment, as were studies conducted in different populations who had a similar constellation of symptoms. The generalizability of studies of nonveterans to veterans is not known.

The best available evidence from studies of treatment for symptoms of CMI and related and comorbid conditions demonstrates that many veterans who have CMI may benefit from such medications as selective serotonin reuptake inhibitors and serotonin norepinephrine reuptake inhibitors and cognitive behavioral therapy. On the basis of the evidence reviewed, the committee cannot recommend any specific therapy as a set treatment for veterans who have CMI. However, for the reasons outlined below, the committee believes that a "one-size-fits-all" approach is not effective for managing veterans who have CMI and that individualized health care management plans are necessary. The condition is complex and not well understood, and it will require more than simply treating veterans with a set protocol of interventions.

> **Recommendation 8-1. The Department of Veterans Affairs should implement a systemwide, integrated, multimodal, long-term management approach to manage veterans who have chronic multisymptom illness.**

VA already has several programs—for example, postdeployment patient-aligned care teams (PD-PACTs), Specialty Care Access Network-Extension for Community Healthcare Outcomes (SCAN-ECHO) programs, and the War-Related Illness and Injury Study Center (WRIISC) program—that could be used to effectively manage veterans who have CMI. However, the programs have not been consistently implemented through the VA health care system. Furthermore, the programs have not been adequately evaluated to learn about their strengths and weaknesses so that changes can be made to improve the quality of care.

Improving Care for Veterans Who Have Chronic Multisymptom Illness

The first step in providing care for veterans who have CMI is to identify them and to move them into VA's health care system so that they can receive proper care for their CMI and any common comorbidities.

> Recommendation 8-2. The Department of Veterans Affairs (VA) should commit the necessary resources to ensure that veterans complete a comprehensive health examination immediately upon separation from active duty. The results should become part of a veteran's health record and should be made available to every clinician caring for the veteran, whether in or outside the VA health care system. Coordination of care, focused on transition in care, is essential for all veterans to ensure quality, patient safety, and the best health outcomes. Any veteran who has chronic multisymptom illness should be able to complete a comprehensive health examination.

> Recommendation 8-3. The Department of Veterans Affairs should include in its electronic health record a "pop-up" screen to prompt clinicians to ask questions about whether a patient has symptoms consistent with the committee's definition of chronic multisymptom illness.

Once a veteran has been identified as having CMI and has entered the VA health care system, the next step is to provide comprehensive care for the veteran, not only for CMI but also for any comorbid conditions. VA has developed multiple clinical practice guidelines (CPGs) for medically unexplained symptoms and common comorbidities and conditions with shared symptoms; however, there is anecdotal evidence that simply adhering to multiple CPGs often is not effective for managing chronic conditions with multiple morbidities such as CMI and can result in incomplete care and increase the likelihood of overtreatment and adverse side effects. Rather, a unique personal care plan for each veteran is required for effective management of the health of veterans who have CMI.

VA's PD-PACTs, which use a team approach to providing coordinated, comprehensive, integrated care, should be able to provide care for veterans who have CMI if properly implemented. The move to the PACT model of care is relatively recent in VA's health care system, and implementation efforts are ongoing.

Recommendation 8-4. The Department of Veterans Affairs (VA) should develop patient-aligned care teams (PACTs) specifically for veterans who have chronic multisymptom illness (CMI; that is, CMI-PACTs) or CMI clinic days in existing PACTs at larger facilities, such as VA medical centers. A needs assessment should be conducted to determine what expertise is necessary to include in a CMI-PACT.

Recommendation 8-5. The Department of Veterans Affairs should commit the resources needed to ensure that patient-aligned care teams have the time and skills required to meet the needs of veterans who have chronic multisymptom illness as specified in the veterans' integrated personal care plans, that the adequacy of time for clinical encounters is measured routinely, and that clinical case loads are adjusted in response to the data generated by measurements. Data from patient experience-of-care surveys are essential to assist in determining needed adjustments.

Recommendation 8-6. The Department of Veterans Affairs should use patient-aligned care teams (PACTs) that have been demonstrated to be centers of excellence as examples so that other PACTs can build on their experiences.

To address the challenges of bringing care to veterans who lack easy access to VA medical centers, VA adopted SCAN-ECHO programs in 2010. SCAN-ECHO programs are being developed to bring specialty care to veterans who live in rural and other underserved areas. The SCAN-ECHO programs work by connecting clinicians who have expertise in particular specialties through video technology to provide case-based consultation and didactics to isolated primary care clinicians who would otherwise not have access to care for their patients.

Another VA program is the WRIISC program, which was established in 2001 to serve combat veterans who had unexplained illnesses. Veterans are generally referred to a WRIISC (there are three nationwide) by their clinicians when they are not improving and further local expertise is not available. Veterans in WRIISCs are evaluated by a multidisciplinary team that conducts a comprehensive health assessment and formulates a comprehensive personal care plan aimed at managing symptoms and improving functional health. Although WRIISCs have been in place for more than a decade, the committee does not have information on awareness of the program among the teams of professionals caring for veterans who have CMI or among the veterans themselves. Information also is lacking on the effectiveness of the program.

Recommendation 8-7. The Department of Veterans Affairs (VA) should develop a process for evaluating awareness among teams of professionals and veterans of its programs for managing veterans who have chronic multisymptom illness, including patient-aligned care teams (PACTs), specialty care access networks (SCANs), and war-related illness and injury study centers (WRIISCs); for providing education where necessary; and for measuring outcomes to determine whether the programs have been successfully implemented and are improving care. Furthermore, VA should take steps to improve coordination of care among PACTs, SCANs, and WRIISCs so that veterans can transition smoothly across these programs.

Dissemination of Information

Many opportunities exist for VA to disseminate information about CMI to clinicians. A major determinant of VA's ability to manage veterans who have CMI is the training of clinicians and teams of professionals in providing care for these patients.

Recommendation 8-8. The Department of Veterans Affairs (VA) should provide resources for and designate "chronic multisymptom illness champions" at each VA medical center. The champions should be integrated into the care system (for example, the patient-aligned care teams) to ensure clear communication and coordination among clinicians.

The champions should be incentivized (for example, by professional advancement and recognition and value-based payment), be given adequate time for office visits with patients who have CMI, have knowledge about the array of therapeutic options that might be useful for treating CMI, have ready access to a team of other clinicians for consultation, and have training in communication skills. Smaller VA facilities, such as community-based outreach clinics, can benefit from CMI champions. For example, the SCAN-ECHO model can be used so that clinicians in community-based outreach clinics or even civilian community-based clinics can contact a CMI champion for expert consultation.

In addition to using CMI champions to train clinicians about CMI, learning networks have been found to be effective tools for disseminating information. Continuous exchange of information among learning networks can lead to improved quality of care. The networks offer a supportive environment for learning skills informally, role models, and a benchmark for an appropriate environment for adopting new practice guidelines.

Recommendation 8-9. The Department of Veterans Affairs (VA) should develop learning, or peer, networks to introduce new information, norms, and skills related to managing veterans who have chronic multi-symptom illness. Because many veterans receive care outside the VA health care system, clinicians in private practice should be offered the opportunity to be included in the learning networks and VA should have a specific focus on community outreach.

Effective patient–clinician communication and coordination of care are crucial for managing veterans who have CMI and are the foundation of patient-centered care and decision making. They are essential for managing such patients successfully.

Recommendation 8-10. The Department of Veterans Affairs should provide required education and training for its clinicians in communicating effectively with and coordinating the care of veterans who have unexplained conditions, such as chronic multisymptom illness.

Improving Data Collection and Quality

As the committee conducted its assessment of treatments for CMI and of how this condition is managed in the VA health care system, it identified gaps in data on performance measurement. To assist VA in improving outcomes and ultimately to improve the quality of care that the VA health care system provides, the committee offers the following recommendation.

Recommendation 8-11. The Department of Veterans Affairs (VA) should provide the resources needed to expand its data collection efforts to include a national system for the robust capture, aggregation, and analysis of data on the structures, processes, and outcomes of care delivery and on the satisfaction with care among patients who have chronic multisymptom illness so that gaps in clinical care can be evaluated, strategies for improvement can be planned, long-term outcomes of treatment can be assessed, and this information can be disseminated to VA health care facilities.

Research Recommendations

The committee's research recommendations are in two categories: treatments for CMI and research needs related to program evaluation.

Treatments for Chronic Multisymptom Illness. Many of the studies of treatments for CMI reviewed by the committee had methodologic flaws that limited their usefulness for the committee's evaluation.

Recommendation 8-12. Future studies funded and conducted by the Department of Veterans Affairs to assess treatments for chronic multi-symptom illness should adhere to the methodologic and reporting guidelines for clinical trials, including appropriate elements (problem–patient–population, intervention, comparison, and outcome of interest) to frame the research question, extended follow-up, active comparators (such as standard of care therapies), and consistent, standardized, validated instruments for measuring outcomes.

Examples of methodologic and reporting guidelines include those set forth by such organizations as the Agency for Healthcare Research and Quality and the Institute of Medicine and in such other efforts as the Preferred Reporting Items for Systematic Reviews and Meta-Analyses statement and the Consolidated Standards of Reporting Trials statement.

On the basis of its assessment of the evidence on treatments for CMI, the committee found that several treatments and treatment approaches may be potentially useful for CMI. However, evidence sufficient to support a conclusion on their effectiveness is lacking.

Recommendation 8-13. The Department of Veterans Affairs should fund and conduct studies of interventions that evidence suggests may hold promise for treatment of chronic multisymptom illness. Specific interventions could include biofeedback, acupuncture, St. John's wort, aerobic exercise, motivational interviewing, and multimodal therapies.

Program Evaluation. As noted above, the committee did not find comprehensive evaluations of VA programs, such as the PACTs, SCAN-ECHO programs, and WRIISCs. Program evaluation—including assessments of structures, processes, and outcomes—is essential if VA is to continually improve its services and research.

Recommendation 8-14. The Department of Veterans Affairs (VA) should apply principles of quality and performance improvement to internally evaluate VA programs and research related to treatments for chronic multisymptom illness (CMI) and overall management of veterans who have CMI. This task can be accomplished using such methods as comparative effectiveness research, translational research, implementation science methods, and health systems research.

REFERENCE

IOM (Institute of Medicine). 2010. *Gulf War and Health, Volume 8: Update of Health Effects of Serving in the Gulf War*. Washington, DC: The National Academies Press. P. 261.

1

Introduction

The purpose of this report is to evaluate and recommend treatments for the array of medically unexplained symptoms—termed chronic multisymptom illness (CMI)—experienced by veterans of the Gulf War. CMI is sometimes referred to as Gulf War syndrome or Gulf War illness. The definition of CMI used in this report is included in Chapter 2.

Throughout modern history, many soldiers returning from combat have experienced postcombat illnesses (Hyams et al., 1996; Jones, 2006; Jones and Wessely, 2005). Efforts to define the illnesses have resulted in descriptive names, such as irritable heart, Da Costa's syndrome, shell shock, combat fatigue, and posttraumatic stress disorder (PTSD). Many soldiers who have postcombat illnesses have long-term unexplained symptoms that cannot now be attributed to any diagnosable pathophysiologic etiology or disease; such symptoms are referred to as medically unexplained. CMI differs from such postcombat illnesses as PTSD that have a defined complex of symptoms (Jones, 2006; Mahoney, 2001; Zavestoski et al., 2004). Soldiers who have CMI often have nonspecific physical symptoms (such as fatigue, joint and muscle pain, and gastrointestinal symptoms) and cognitive symptoms (such as reduced processing speed and memory difficulties) in addition to symptoms that are commonly associated with depression and anxiety.

PRIOR EFFORTS TO ADDRESS CHRONIC MULTISYMPTOM ILLNESS IN GULF WAR VETERANS

In efforts to understand CMI and how to treat for it, substantial resources have been devoted to determining its underlying cause. Government agencies in the United States and elsewhere have pursued or funded ambitious research programs to study CMI (Mahoney, 2001; Zavestoski et al., 2004). Most research on the cause of CMI has focused on environmental toxicants to which military personnel may have been exposed. Those toxicants include a long list of chemical, biologic, and physical agents (Persian Gulf War Veterans Act of 1998, Public Law 277, 105th Cong., October 8, 1998; Veterans Programs Enhancement Act of 1998, Public Law 368, 105th Cong., October 21, 1998). The focus on toxicants may be attributed, at least in part, to "a general fear of toxins spread as a result of modern industrial life" (Jones and Wessely, 2005). Many agents used in combat operation may be harmful to humans, depending on exposure routes and quantities. Concern about health effects of exposure to toxicants during war became ingrained in our culture with the Vietnam War, when a herbicide, Agent Orange, was implicated as a source of serious health problems in veterans and others who were exposed.

The present committee is not the first Institute of Medicine (IOM) committee to evaluate treatments for CMI in Gulf War veterans. In 2001, IOM released a report, *Gulf War Veterans: Treating Symptoms and Syndromes*, which examined how to manage medically unexplained physical symptoms (MUPS; termed CMI in this report) (IOM, 2001). The committee that wrote that report found sparse evidence on treatments for MUPS and so was unable to recommend specific treatments. It did, however, recommend a general approach for the management of patients who had MUPS. That approach included

- Using diagnostic testing and medication only as medically necessary.
- Using appropriate reassurance strategies to comfort patients.
- Setting realistic goals in collaboration with patients.
- Encouraging patients to exercise regularly to improve functioning.
- Encouraging patients to involve their families and friends, if appropriate, in their care.
- Coordinating care among clinicians so that patients do not bounce from specialist to specialist, receive many unnecessary diagnostic procedures, and end up on multiple unnecessary medications.
- Introducing specialty mental health consultation, if needed. ("Most patients with MUPS do not require psychiatric treatment or psychological testing.") (IOM, 2001).

In 2006 and again in 2010, IOM committees reviewed and evaluated the scientific literature on the health status of 1991 Gulf War veterans. Both committees found that veterans of the 1991 Gulf War who had been deployed reported more symptoms than their nondeployed counterparts (IOM, 2006b, 2010a). The later report concluded that there is "sufficient evidence of association between deployment to the Gulf War and chronic multisymptom illness" (p. 210), that "the excess of unexplained medical symptoms reported by deployed Gulf War veterans cannot be reliably ascribed to any known psychiatric disorder" (p. 109), and that the unexplained symptoms might "result from interplay between . . . biological and psychological factors" (p. 260).

A number of IOM reports have examined associations between health outcomes and exposures that military personnel may have been subject to during their service in the 1991 Gulf War—chemical exposures (for example, to combustion products, pesticides, pyridostigmine bromide, sarin, and solvents), biologic exposures (for example, to infectious agents and vaccines), and physical exposures (for example, to depleted uranium) (IOM, 2000, 2003, 2004, 2005, 2006a,b, 2007, 2008, 2010a). In sum, those reports did not find evidence that would support a confident attribution of the array of unexplained symptoms reported by veterans of the 1991 Gulf War to any specific chemical, biologic, or physical exposure.

There is a lack of consensus among expert groups regarding the cause of CMI in 1991 Gulf War veterans. Most experts who have studied the issue have not identified what they consider to be a likely cause of CMI. However, the Department of Veterans Affairs (VA) Research Advisory Committee on Gulf War Veterans' Illness (RAC) conducted a review of the evidence and concluded that Gulf War illness was causally associated with use of pyridostigmine bromide pills and exposure to pesticides used during deployment (RAC, 2008). IOM reviewed the epidemiologic and experimental studies cited in the RAC report and concluded that the evidence was not robust enough to establish a causal relationship between pyridostigmine bromide or pesticides and CMI (IOM, 2010a).

Despite many years of research, there is no consensus among physicians, researchers, and others as to the cause of CMI in 1991 Gulf War veterans, and there is a growing belief that a causal factor or agent may not be identified (IOM, 2010a; Mahoney, 2001). It is also possible that an underlying physiologic abnormality may not be identified. The 2010 IOM committee recommended "a renewed research effort with substantial commitment to well-organized efforts to better identify and treat multisymptom illness in Gulf War veterans" (IOM, 2010a).

THE CHARGE TO THE COMMITTEE

The present study was mandated by Congress in the Veterans Benefits Act of 2010 (Public Law 111-275, October 13, 2010). The law directs the secretary of veterans affairs "to enter into an agreement with the Institute of Medicine of the National Academies to carry out a comprehensive review of the best treatments for CMI in Persian Gulf War veterans and an evaluation of how such treatment approaches could best be disseminated throughout the Department of Veterans Affairs to improve the care and benefits provided to veterans." In August 2011, VA asked that IOM conduct a study to address that charge, and IOM appointed the Committee on Gulf War and Health: Treatment for Chronic Multisymptom Illness. The complete charge to the committee is in Box 1-1. A description of how the committee approached its charge can be found in Chapter 3 and its evaluation of the evidence, conclusions, and recommendations are presented in Chapters 4–8.

BOX 1-1
The Committee's Charge

The Institute of Medicine (IOM) will convene a committee to comprehensively review, evaluate, and summarize the available scientific and medical literature regarding the best treatments for chronic multisymptom illness among Gulf War veterans.

In its evaluation, the committee will look broadly for relevant information. Information sources to pursue could include, but are not limited to

- Published peer-reviewed literature concerning the treatment of multisymptom illness among the 1991 Gulf War veteran population;
- Published peer-reviewed literature concerning treatment of multisymptom illness among Operation Enduring Freedom, Operation Iraqi Freedom, and Operation New Dawn active-duty service members and veterans;
- Published peer-reviewed literature concerning treatment of multisymptom illness among similar populations such as allied military personnel; and
- Published peer-reviewed literature concerning treatment of populations with a similar constellation of symptoms.

In addition to summarizing the available scientific and medical literature regarding the best treatments for chronic multisymptom illness among Gulf War veterans, the IOM will

- Recommend how best to disseminate this information throughout the Department of Veterans Affairs to improve the care and benefits provided to veterans.
- Recommend additional scientific studies and research initiatives to resolve areas of continuing scientific uncertainty.
- Recommend such legislative or administrative action as the IOM deems appropriate in light of the results of its review.

THE GULF WAR VETERAN POPULATION

Veterans are considered to have served in the Gulf War if they were on active military duty in the Southwest Asia theater of military operations during the period from the 1991 Gulf War (Operation Desert Storm) through the Iraq War (Operation Iraqi Freedom and Operation New Dawn) (VA, 2012b). The Gulf War officially began on August 2, 1990, when Iraqi troops invaded Kuwait. US and coalition troops arrived in the theater in January 1991, and combat was over on February 28, 1991. A cease-fire with Iraq was signed in April 1991, and the last US troops participating in the ground war arrived back in the United States in June of that year. During the 1990s, US troops participated in a variety of military activities in the Southwest Asia theater of operation. The United States has not formally declared an end to the Gulf War, and the Iraq War is considered part of the same military mission (VA, 2011). For the purpose of this report, although Afghanistan is not in the Southwest Asia theater of operation, veterans of the Afghanistan War (Operation Enduring Freedom) are included in the Gulf War veteran population. A substantial number of soldiers have served in both the Iraq and Afghanistan theaters of operation. Three populations of Gulf War veterans are referred to in this report: 1991 Gulf War veterans, Iraq War veterans, and Afghanistan War veterans.

About 700,000 military personnel participated in the 1991 Gulf War (VA, 2012a). Estimates of the numbers of 1991 Gulf War veterans who have CMI range from 175,000 to 250,000 (about 25–35% of the 1991 Gulf War veteran population) (IOM, 2010a; RAC, 2008). As noted above and discussed in more detail in later chapters, 1991 Gulf War veterans who have CMI experience a large constellation of symptoms. A number of research studies have been conducted to determine whether those symptoms can be grouped into symptom clusters (see the 2010 IOM report for a summary of the studies), but the research has identified no symptom clusters, or syndromes.

There is evidence that CMI in 1991 Gulf War veterans may not resolve over time. Many of the symptoms reported by veterans of that war are chronic. Ill veterans in general (not only those who have CMI) who were deployed to the gulf in 1991 are more likely than nondeployed veterans who served during the same era to report persistent health problems and to develop new ones (Li et al., 2011). Health outcomes assessed by Li et al. (2011) include chronic fatigue syndrome–like illness, functional impairment, limitation of activities, clinic visits and hospitalizations, and self-perception of health.

As discussed above, Gulf War veterans include military personnel who served in the Iraq war and, for the purpose of this report, the Afghanistan war, in addition to those who served in the 1991 war. As of September

2011, 2.6 million military personnel have been deployed to Iraq or Afghanistan (GAO, 2011).

Deployments to the Iraq and Afghanistan war theaters differ somewhat from deployments to the 1991 Gulf War. Women make up about 11% of US military personnel who have served in Iraq and Afghanistan compared with about 7% in the 1991 Gulf War (IOM, 2010a,b). Nearly one-fourth of military personnel who have served in Iraq and Afghanistan have been from the National Guard and reserves compared with about 17% in the 1991 Gulf War (IOM, 2010a,b). National Guard and reserve personnel are substantially older than active-duty personnel; for example, 73.6% of reserve officers are over 35 years old compared with 44.2% of active-duty officers (IOM, 2010b). Military personnel in the Iraq and Afghanistan wars have been exposed to more hostile fire, including blasts from improvised explosive devices. Their deployments are longer than those in the 1991 Gulf War, and repeated deployments are common. Personnel who have at least one prior deployment are more likely to screen positive for PTSD and major depression and to report chronic pain than those who have no prior deployments (Kline et al., 2010).

Three health conditions often are associated with service in the Iraq and Afghanistan wars: PTSD, traumatic brain injury (TBI), and chronic pain. Lew et al. (2009) reviewed medical records of 340 Iraq and Afghanistan war veterans at a VA polytrauma center and found that the prevalence of PTSD was 68.2%, of persistent postconcussive symptoms from TBI 66.8%, and of chronic pain 81.5%. A substantial number of those veterans—42.1%—had all three conditions. Other studies have also reported high rates of that triad of conditions (Reisinger et al., 2012; Walker et al., 2010). Symptoms reported by Iraq and Afghanistan war veterans include headaches, chronic pain (particularly lower back and joint pain), sleep disturbances, fatigue, irritability, and concentration, attention, and memory problems (Walker et al., 2010). Many symptoms experienced by Iraq and Afghanistan war veterans overlap with those experienced by 1991 Gulf War veterans.

GULF WAR VETERANS' EXPERIENCES WITH DIAGNOSIS OF AND TREATMENT FOR CHRONIC MULTISYMPTOM ILLNESS

During the 1991 Gulf War and on returning to the United States after deployment, ill veterans have sought help for the diagnosis of and treatment for their CMI. Many were seen initially by clinicians at VA facilities but became frustrated because VA clinicians diagnosed psychologic conditions (for example, depression, anxiety disorders, stress-related complaints, and somatoform disorders) (Shriver and Waskul, 2006; Swoboda, 2006). Often, they received no diagnosis at all (Zavestoski et al., 2004) or received many diagnoses and were confused by what they "officially" had (Furey, 2012).

In some cases, the veterans sought answers to their health problems from private clinicians, often at great personal financial expense.

Losing trust in medical professionals, veterans have also searched for information about their symptoms and potential diagnoses and treatments through the Internet, medical books and articles, newspapers, their peers, and other sources (Swoboda, 2006). An analysis of veterans' Internet use related to CMI suggests that their primary means of Internet communication is discussion boards, although blogs (including microblogs), Facebook, and media-sharing are also used (Furey, 2012). Their searches sometimes have led them to alternative medical treatments, such as unconventional diets, detoxification, vitamins, physical and manipulative therapies, religious and metaphysical practices, and "New Age" and self-improvement philosophies (Furey, 2012; Swoboda, 2006).

Because those who are ill do not have a disease with a distinct etiology, veterans of the 1991 Gulf War believe that the legitimacy of their illness is often called into question by clinicians, family members, friends, and others (Shriver and Waskul, 2006). The stress caused by the necessity to prove repeatedly that they are ill can add to the veterans' health problems by creating anxiety, which in turn may exacerbate the veterans' symptoms (Zavestoski et al., 2004).

Some ill 1991 Gulf War veterans, believing that they are being given wrong diagnoses and are being inadequately treated by clinicians, view themselves as "victims of an entrenched medical discourse that makes it difficult for many practitioners to recognize new patterns of illness" (Swoboda, 2006, p. 247). They are left feeling distrustful of and betrayed by the health care system (Furey, 2012). Therefore, it is not surprising that a different approach to managing veterans who have CMI has been proposed (Mahoney, 2001; Zavestoski et al., 2004). Mahoney (2001) stated that clinicians should approach CMI with "a person-centered rather than a disease-centered model of care that allows patients more control over their diagnoses and treatment plans, that helps patients understand that the word psychosomatic is not pejorative, and that concentrates less on finding the origin of disease than on treating its symptoms" (p. 581).

ORGANIZATION OF THIS REPORT

The committee's work is presented in seven additional chapters. Chapter 2 explains the terminology surrounding CMI and how the term is used by the committee. It also covers what is known about CMI (for example, the understanding of its course) and why the committee believes that it is appropriate to evaluate the literature on CMI in populations other than Gulf War veterans as part of its analysis. Chapter 3 describes how the committee approached its charge, including its strategy for assessing treatments for CMI. Chapter 4 summarizes the evidence on treatments for CMI and the committee's evaluation of it. Chapter 5 discusses evidence-based treatment practices for conditions that either have overlapping symptoms with CMI or present comorbidly with CMI (for example, chronic fatigue syndrome, fibromyalgia, irritable bowel syndrome, depression, and anxiety). Chapter 6 describes how the way in which clinicians engage with their patients can affect the course of CMI. Chapter 7 provides information on VA's current model of care for veterans who have CMI and describes alternative models of care and how they may be implemented by VA health care system. Finally, Chapter 8 presents the committee's recommendations. Brief biographies of the committee members are in Appendix A, a discussion of possible factors underlying the symptoms of CMI in Appendix B, and examples of ineffective and effective clinician–patient discussions in Appendix C.

REFERENCES

Furey, P. 2012 (unpublished). *Analysis of the Social Media Discussion of Chronic Multi-symptom Illness in Veterans of the Iraq and Afghanistan Wars.* Analysis commissioned by the Committee on Gulf War and Health: Treatment of Chronic Multisymptom Illness, Institute of Medicine, Washington, DC.

GAO (Government Accountability Office). 2011. *VA Mental Health: Number of Veterans Receiving Care, Barriers Faced, and Efforts to Increase Access.* Washington, DC: GAO 12-12.

Hyams, K. C., F. S. Wignall, and R. Roswell. 1996. War syndromes and their evaluation: From the US Civil War to the Persian Gulf War. *Annals of Internal Medicine* 125(5):398-405.

IOM (Institute of Medicine). 2000. *Gulf War and Health, Volume 1: Depleted Uranium, Pyridostigmine Bromide, Sarin, Vaccines.* Washington, DC: National Academy Press.

IOM. 2001. *Gulf War Veterans: Treating Symptoms and Syndromes, The Compass Series.* Washington, DC: National Academy Press.

IOM. 2003. *Gulf War and Health, Volume 2: Insecticides and Solvents.* Washington, DC: The National Academies Press.

IOM. 2004. *Gulf War and Health: Updated Literature Review of Sarin.* Washington, DC: The National Academies Press.

IOM. 2005. *Gulf War and Health, Volume 3: Fuels, Combustion Products, and Propellants.* Washington, DC: The National Academies Press.

IOM. 2006a. *Amyotrophic Lateral Sclerosis in Veterans: Review of the Scientific Literature.* Washington, DC: The National Academies Press.

IOM. 2006b. *Gulf War and Health, Volume 4: Health Effects of Serving in the Gulf War.* Washington, DC: The National Academies Press.

IOM. 2007. *Gulf War and Health, Volume 5: Infectious Diseases.* Washington, DC: The National Academies Press.

IOM. 2008. *Gulf War and Health: Updated Literature Review of Depleted Uranium.* Washington, DC: The National Academies Press.

IOM. 2010a. *Gulf War and Health, Volume 8: Update of Health Effects of Serving in the Gulf War.* Washington, DC: The National Academies Press.

IOM. 2010b. *Returning Home from Iraq and Afghanistan: Preliminary Assessment of Readjustment Needs of Veterans, Service Members, and Their Families.* Washington, DC: The National Academies Press.

Jones, E. 2006. Historical approaches to post-combat disorders. *Philosophical Transactions of the Royal Society of London—Series B: Biological Sciences* 361(1468):533-542.

Jones, E., and S. Wessely. 2005. War syndromes: The impact of culture on medically unexplained symptoms. *Medical History* 49(1):55-78.

Kline, A., M. Falca-Dodson, B. Sussner, D. S. Ciccone, H. Chandler, L. Callahan, and M. Losonczy. 2010. Effects of repeated deployment to Iraq and Afghanistan on the health of New Jersey Army national guard troops: Implications for military readiness. *American Journal of Public Health* 100(2):276-283.

Lew, H. L., J. D. Otis, C. Tun, R. D. Kerns, M. E. Clark, and D. X. Cifu. 2009. Prevalence of chronic pain, posttraumatic stress disorder, and persistent postconcussive symptoms in OIF/OEF veterans: Polytrauma clinical triad. *Journal of Rehabilitation Research and Development* 46(6):697-702.

Li, B., C. M. Mahan, H. K. Kang, S. A. Eisen, and C. C. Engel. 2011. Longitudinal health study of US 1991 Gulf War veterans: Changes in health status at 10-year follow-up. *American Journal of Epidemiology* 174(7):761-768.

Mahoney, D. B. 2001. A normative construction of Gulf War syndrome. *Perspectives in Biology & Medicine* 44(4):575-583.

RAC (Research Advisory Committee on Gulf War Veterans' Illnesses). 2008. *Scientific Findings and Recommendations.* Washington, DC: RAC.

Reisinger, H. S., S. C. Hunt, A. L. Burgo-Black, and M. A. Agarwal. 2012. A population approach to mitigating the long-term health effects of combat deployments. *Preventing Chronic Disease* 9:E54.

Shriver, T. E., and D. D. Waskul. 2006. Managing the uncertainties of Gulf War illness: The challenges of living with contested illness. *Symbolic Interaction* 29(4):465-486.

Swoboda, D. A. 2006. The social construction of contested illness legitimacy: A grounded theory analysis. *Qualitative Research in Psychology* 3(3):233-251.

VA (Department of Veterans Affairs). 2011. *Gulf War Era Veterans Report: Pre-9/11 (August 2, 1990 to September 10, 2001).* Washington, DC: VA.

VA. 2012a. *About the Gulf War.* http://www.publichealth.va.gov/exposures/gulfwar/basics.asp (accessed May 8, 2012).

VA. 2012b. *Gulf War Service.* http://www.publichealth.va.gov/exposures/gulfwar/military-service.asp (accessed May 18, 2012).

Walker, R. L., M. E. Clark, and S. H. Sanders. 2010. The "postdeployment multi-symptom disorder": An emerging syndrome in need of a new treatment paradigm. *Psychological Services* 7(3):136-147.

Zavestoski, S., P. Brown, S. McCormick, B. Mayer, M. D'Ottavi, and J. C. Lucove. 2004. Patient activism and the struggle for diagnosis: Gulf War illnesses and other medically unexplained physical symptoms in the US. *Social Science & Medicine* 58(1):161-175.

2

Characterizing Chronic Multisymptom Illness

Before evaluating treatments for chronic multisymptom illness (CMI), the committee defined it. The terminology surrounding CMI can be confusing, and it is inconsistently defined in the literature. This chapter covers the following issues:

- Terms used to characterize conditions that are similar to CMI. These terms sometimes are used interchangeably and at other times have distinct meanings.
- The committee's definition of CMI.
- What is known about CMI in the general, military, and veteran populations.
- The goals of treating for CMI.

TERMINOLOGY

The term *chronic multisymptom illness* was first used to describe chronic unexplained symptoms in Air Force veterans of the 1991 Gulf War (Fukuda et al., 1998). CMI was defined as the report by a veteran of one or more chronic unexplained symptoms (present for 6 months or longer) in at least two of the following categories:

- Fatigue.
- Mood and cognition (symptoms of feeling depressed, difficulty in remembering or concentrating, feeling moody, feeling anxious, trouble in finding words, or difficulty in sleeping).

- Musculoskeletal (symptoms of joint pain, joint stiffness, or muscle pain).

Because the study was funded and conducted by the Centers for Disease Control and Prevention (CDC), that characterization is often referred to as CDC's case definition of CMI.

Before 1998, the terms *Gulf War syndrome, Gulf War veterans' illness, unexplained illness*, and *undiagnosed illness* were used interchangeably to describe chronic unexplained symptoms in veterans of the 1991 Gulf War. Earlier committees of the Institute of Medicine (IOM) found no evidence of a specific symptom complex (or syndrome) that was peculiar to deployed Gulf War veterans (IOM, 2006, 2010).

Reports of chronic unexplained symptoms are not peculiar to Gulf War veterans; this phenomenon has been documented in military personnel throughout modern history (Hyams et al., 1996; IOM, 2010; Jones, 2006). Before World War I, such chronic unexplained symptoms as fatigue, shortness of breath, and chest pain were referred to as *irritable heart, soldier's heart, Da Costa's syndrome*, and others. Other terms associated with the adverse effects of combat experience on health and well-being include *shell shock* (World War I), *psychoneurosis* (World War II and the Korean War), and *post-Vietnam syndrome*, later identified as posttraumatic stress disorder (PTSD) (Jones, 2006). A cluster analysis of common symptoms in veterans from 1900 to the 1991 Gulf War did not reveal a unique set of symptoms that were associated with each war (Jones and Wessely, 2005; Jones et al., 2002). However, veterans of the 1991 Gulf War have reported more cases of chronic medically unexplained symptoms than veterans of prior conflicts (Hunt, 2012).

Chronic unexplained symptoms are common in civilians. Such terms as *medically unexplained symptoms, medically unexplained physical symptoms, somatoform disorders* (for example, *somatization disorder, undifferentiated somatoform disorder*, and *pain disorder*), and *functional somatic syndromes* are often used to describe the disorders of civilians who have chronic unexplained symptoms. The common thread among the terms is that symptoms experienced by patients cannot be explained as pathologically defined, or organic, disease (Sharpe and Carson, 2001). Such syndromes as irritable bowel syndrome (IBS), chronic fatigue syndrome (CFS, also called myalgic encephalomyelitis), and fibromyalgia often are included in this group of unexplained illnesses, as are chronic unexplained symptoms that do not meet case definitions for IBS, CFS, fibromyalgia, and other functional somatic syndromes that have specified diagnostic criteria.

THE COMMITTEE'S WORKING DEFINITION OF
CHRONIC MULTISYMPTOM ILLNESS

To approach its task, the committee first developed a working definition of CMI. It began by considering the CDC definition described above. Fukuda et al. (1998) arrived at their case definition for CMI by using both a statistical approach called factor analysis and a clinical approach in which symptoms had to be reported for at least 6 months by at least 25% of 1991 Gulf War Air Force veterans enrolled in the study and by deployed veterans at least 2.5 times more often than by nondeployed military personnel. Three categories of symptoms were included in their case definition: fatigue, mood and cognition, and musculoskeletal. Other types of reported symptoms—including gastrointestinal, respiratory, and neurologic—did not meet the threshold for the case definition. The committee decided to broaden its working definition to include respiratory, gastrointestinal, and neurologic symptoms because previous IOM reports found that these types of symptoms were commonly reported by 1991 Gulf War veterans (IOM, 2006, 2010). As suggested in the 1995 IOM report *Health Consequences of Service During the Persian Gulf War: Initial Findings and Recommendations for Immediate Action*, a reasonable case definition of CMI is necessary for VA hospitals to identify veterans who are eligible for care for their symptoms (IOM, 1995). Correctly identifying a health condition may improve patient care and avoid unnecessary tests (Wegman et al., 1997).

CMI is a complex, amorphous condition and its case definition may change as new scientific information emerges. For the purpose of this report, the committee defined CMI as follows:

> The presence of a spectrum of chronic symptoms experienced for 6 months or longer in at least two of six categories—fatigue, mood and cognition, musculoskeletal, gastrointestinal, respiratory, and neurologic—that may overlap with but are not fully captured by known syndromes (such as IBS, CFS, and fibromyalgia) or other diagnoses.

It is important to note that the committee's definition does not include syndromes that have well-defined diagnostic criteria, such as IBS, CFS, and fibromyalgia. However, because of the shared symptoms, effective therapies for those defined syndromes may be beneficial to patients who have CMI. Chapter 5 of this report explores the evidence that supports therapies for the other syndromes and discusses the possible application of the therapies for managing CMI.

As discussed in Chapter 7, the Department of Veterans Affairs (VA) provides disability compensation for CMI associated with Gulf War service without regard to cause (38 CFR Sec. 3.317).

CHRONIC MULTISYMPTOM ILLNESS IN
CIVILIAN AND VETERAN POPULATIONS

Most people experience some unexplained symptoms—symptoms that cannot be attributed to any organic cause—during their lifetimes; unexplained symptoms can account for one-fourth to half of all patient visits to primary care clinicians (Burton, 2003; Janca et al., 2006; Kroenke et al., 1990). Patients who have unexplained symptoms are seen in primary care practices and in medical specialty practices (for example, gynecology, gastroenterology, and rheumatology) (Nimnuan et al., 2001).

However, some people have such symptoms repeatedly. In general, chronic medically unexplained symptoms (lasting 6 months or more) remain unexplained and unresolved. One study reported that the symptoms of almost 60% of patients who had unexplained symptoms remained unexplained over a 12-month period (Koch et al., 2009). The longer the patient had the symptoms before presentation, the poorer the long-term prognosis.

A comprehensive review of the literature on unexplained symptoms found that "many patients with MUPS [medically unexplained physical symptoms] have no definite psychological illness" (Burton, 2003, p. 235). Others have concluded that unexplained symptoms are likely to be multifactorial and include physiologic, psychologic, and social factors (Sharpe and Mayou, 2004).

Numerous studies have examined the symptoms reported by veterans of the 1991 Gulf War. They have been summarized and evaluated by IOM (2006, 2010) and will not be reexamined here. Briefly, although symptom reporting was inconsistent among studies and no single symptom complex, or syndrome, was identified, deployed 1991 Gulf War veterans reported increased prevalence of fatigue, nervous system symptoms, respiratory symptoms, chronic musculoskeletal pain, gastrointestinal symptoms, mood and cognitive abnormalities, and sleep disturbance compared with nondeployed 1991 Gulf War–era veterans.

Estimates of the prevalence of CMI among deployed 1991 Gulf War veterans indicate that CMI is twice as common in deployed veterans as in nondeployed 1991 Gulf War–era veterans. In one study, 45% of Air Force veterans of the 1991 Gulf War met the criteria for CMI compared with 15% of nondeployed 1991 Gulf War–era veterans (Fukuda et al., 1998). In a separate study that used the same definition of CMI as Fukuda et al. (1998), the prevalence of CMI was 29% among deployed 1991 Gulf War veterans and 16% among nondeployed 1991 Gulf War–era veterans 10 years after the end of the Gulf War (Blanchard et al., 2006). In these studies, CMI was statistically significantly associated with service in the Gulf War, enlisted rank, female sex, and smoking (Fukuda et al., 1998) and prewar depression and anxiety (Blanchard et al., 2006). A 10-year follow-up study that tracked the health of 1991 Gulf War veterans found that deployed veterans continued to report persistently poorer health than nondeployed veterans (Li et al., 2011). It was found that the deployed veterans were less likely to improve and more likely to experience a new onset of adverse health outcomes, including fatigue, than their nondeployed counterparts. VA continues to conduct research to follow the health of the 1991 Gulf War veterans (VA, 2012b). The most recent survey in the series began in May 2012 and includes questions related to CMI.

Information about the prevalence of medically unexplained symptoms in veterans of the Iraq and Afghanistan wars is sparse. The most common health outcomes reported in the literature associated with service in the Iraq and Afghanistan wars are PTSD, mild traumatic brain injury, and pain (Walker et al., 2010). One study reported that the prevalence of that triad of conditions in veterans of the Iraq and Afghanistan wars who were seen in a VA polytrauma clinic was 42% (Lew et al., 2009).

Veterans of the Iraq and Afghanistan wars report a number of symptoms (see Box 2-1). Some—sleep disturbance; concentration, attention,

---

BOX 2-1
Symptoms and Related Functional Impairment
Reported by Veterans of Operation Iraqi Freedom,
Operation Enduring Freedom, and Operation New Dawn

- Sleep disturbance
- Low frustration tolerance and irritability
- Concentration, attention, and memory problems
- Fatigue
- Headaches
- Musculoskeletal disorders
- Affective disturbance
- Apathy
- Personality change
- Substance misuse (including opioid misuse)
- Activity avoidance and kinesiophobia
- Hypervigilance
- Employment or school difficulties
- Relationship conflict

SOURCE: Adapted from Walker et al., 2010. Original print available in the public domain.

and memory problems; fatigue; headaches; and musculoskeletal pain problems—also have been reported by 1991 Gulf War veterans. Walker et al. (2010) have proposed that the presentation of symptoms in veterans of the Iraq and Afghanistan wars be called "postdeployment multisymptom disorder." One of the more common diagnoses among veterans of the Iraq and Afghanistan wars (nearly 52% of the veterans) is symptoms, signs, and ill-defined conditions (that is, conditions that do not have an immediately obvious cause or isolated laboratory-test abnormalities) (VA, 2012a).

Among 335 responses to the 1-year postdeployment assessment completed by National Guard and Army service members participating in the HEROES study, 57.2% met the definition of CMI proposed by Fukuda et al. (1998). Risk factors associated with CMI identified from this cohort include combat exposure, number of stressful deployment experiences, PTSD symptoms, predeployment stressful life events, and severe nonspecific physical symptoms before deployment (McAndrew et al., 2012).

VETERAN VS CIVILIAN POPULATIONS

In this report, the committee uses, as part of its evidence base, studies conducted in populations other than Gulf War veterans. As noted above, experiencing chronic unexplained symptoms is not peculiar to Gulf War veterans and in fact is common in the general population.

Veterans of the 1991 Gulf War may have a higher prevalence of unexplained symptoms than veterans of previous conflicts (Hunt, 2012), but the types of symptoms appear to be consistent with the types experienced by veterans of other wars and by civilians.

There are important differences between studies of civilians and studies of veterans. For example, in studies of unexplained symptoms in civilians, the samples tend to be mostly white women of middle age; only about 7% of military personnel in the 1991 Gulf War were women, and the overall mean age was 28 years.

MANAGING VS CURING CHRONIC MULTISYMPTOM ILLNESS

It is important to continue to describe, classify, and explain CMI. Many clinicians, patients, and family members are understandably focused on finding a specific etiology and cure. In the meantime, veterans who have CMI and the clinicians who care for them have clamored for assistance in improving function and outcomes of those who have the condition. Veterans must find a way to live productive lives in spite of their CMI, and clinicians must offer care for patients who have conditions that remain unexplained. The experience with medically unexplained symptoms and similar syndromes in the general population suggests that although a cure for CMI may be elusive, effective management is possible. Many patients are deprived of the benefits of an organized, systematic approach to the clinical management of CMI. The present committee's goal is to provide an organized, systematic approach to management for veterans who have CMI.

REFERENCES

Blanchard, M. S., S. A. Eisen, R. Alpern, J. Karlinsky, R. Toomey, D. J. Reda, F. M. Murphy, L. W. Jackson, and H. K. Kang. 2006. Chronic multisymptom illness complex in Gulf War I veterans 10 years later. *American Journal of Epidemiology* 163(1):66-75.

Burton, C. 2003. Beyond somatisation: A review of the understanding and treatment of medically unexplained physical symptoms (MUPS). *British Journal of General Practice* 53(488):231-239.

Fukuda, K., R. Nisenbaum, G. Stewart, W. W. Thompson, L. Robin, R. M. Washko, D. L. Noah, D. H. Barrett, B. Randall, B. L. Herwaldt, A. C. Mawle, and W. C. Reeves. 1998. Chronic multisymptom illness affecting Air Force veterans of the Gulf War. *Journal of the American Medical Association* 280(11):981-988.

Hunt, S. C. 2012. *VA Approaches to the Management of Chronic Multi-symptom Illness in Gulf War I Veterans.* Presentation at the Third Committee Meeting, April 12, 2012, Irvine, CA.

Hyams, K. C., F. S. Wignall, and R. Roswell. 1996. War syndromes and their evaluation: From the US Civil War to the Persian Gulf War. *Annals of Internal Medicine* 125(5):398-405.

IOM (Institute of Medicine). 1995. *Health Consequences of Service During the Persian Gulf War: Initial Findings and Recommendations for Immediate Action.* Washington, DC: National Academy Press.

IOM. 2006. *Gulf War and Health, Volume 4: Health Effects of Serving in the Gulf War.* Washington, DC: The National Academies Press.

IOM. 2010. *Gulf War and Health, Volume 8: Update of Health Effects of Serving in the Gulf War.* Washington, DC: The National Academies Press.

Janca, A., M. Isaac, and J. Ventouras. 2006. Towards better understanding and management of somatoform disorders. *International Review of Psychiatry* 18(1):5-12.

Jones, E. 2006. Historical approaches to post-combat disorders. *Philosophical Transactions of the Royal Society of London—Series B: Biological Sciences* 361(1468):533-542.

Jones, E., and S. Wessely. 2005. War syndromes: The impact of culture on medically unexplained symptoms. *Medical History* 49(1):55-78.

Jones, E., R. Hodgins-Vermaas, H. McCartney, B. Everitt, C. Beech, D. Poynter, I. Palmer, K. Hyams, and S. Wessely. 2002. Post-combat syndromes from the Boer War to the Gulf War: A cluster analysis of their nature and attribution. [erratum appears in BMJ 324(7334):397]. *British Medical Journal* 324(7333):321-324.

Koch, H., M. A. van Bokhoven, P. J. E. Bindels, T. van der Weijden, G. J. Dinant, and G. ter Riet. 2009. The course of newly presented unexplained complaints in general practice patients: A prospective cohort study. *Family Practice* 26(6):455-465.

Kroenke, K., M. E. Arrington, and A. D. Mangelsdorff. 1990. The prevalence of symptoms in medical outpatients and the adequacy of therapy. *Archives of Internal Medicine* 150(8):1685-1689.

Lew, H. L., J. D. Otis, C. Tun, R. D. Kerns, M. E. Clark, and D. X. Cifu. 2009. Prevalence of chronic pain, posttraumatic stress disorder, and persistent postconcussive symptoms in OIF/OEF veterans: Polytrauma clinical triad. *Journal of Rehabilitation Research and Development* 46(6):697-702.

Li, B., C. M. Mahan, H. K. Kang, S. A. Eisen, and C. C. Engel. 2011. Longitudinal health study of US 1991 Gulf War veterans: Changes in health status at 10-year follow-up. *American Journal of Epidemiology* 174(7):761-768.

McAndrew, L. M., H. K. Chandler, E. A. D'Andrea, G. Lang, C. Engel, and K. S. Quigley. 2012. *Chronic Multisymptom Illness: An Unrecognized Public Health Concern Among OEF/OIF Veterans.* Paper presented at HSR&D/QUERI National Conference 2012, National Harbor, MD. http://www.hsrd.research.va.gov/meetings/2012/abstract-display. cfm?RecordID=590 (accessed September 12, 2012).

Nimnuan, C., M. Hotopf, and S. Wessely. 2001. Medically unexplained symptoms: An epidemiological study in seven specialities. *Journal of Psychosomatic Research* 51(1):361-367.

Sharpe, M., and A. Carson. 2001. "Unexplained" somatic symptoms, functional syndromes, and somatization: Do we need a paradigm shift? *Annals of Internal Medicine* 134(9 Pt 2):926-930.

Sharpe, M., and R. Mayou. 2004. Somatoform disorders: A help or hindrance to good patient care? *British Journal of Psychiatry* 184:465-467.

VA (Department of Veterans Affairs). 2012a. *Analysis of VA Health Care Utilization Among Operation Enduring Freedom (OEF), Operation Iraqi Freedom (OIF), and Operation New Dawn (OND) Veterans.* http://www.publichealth.va.gov/docs/epidemiology/ healthcare-utilization-report-fy2012-qtr2.pdf (accessed September 12, 2012).

VA. 2012b. *Gulf War Follow-Up Study.* http://www.publichealth.va.gov/epidemiology/studies/ gulf-war-follow-up.asp (accessed September 12, 2012).

Walker, R. L., M. E. Clark, and S. H. Sanders. 2010. The "postdeployment multi-symptom disorder": An emerging syndrome in need of a new treatment paradigm. *Psychological Services* 7(3):136-147.

Wegman, D. H., N. F. Woods, and J. C. Bailar. 1997. Invited commentary: How would we know a Gulf War syndrome if we saw one? *American Journal of Epidemiology* 146(9):704-711; discussion 712.

3

Methods

To respond to its charge (see Chapter 1), the committee needed a multi-pronged approach. This chapter describes the committee's methods.

The committee conducted a systematic review to evaluate the scientific literature on therapies to eliminate or alleviate the symptoms associated with chronic multisymptom illness (CMI). Details on the methods of the review are included below, and the results of the review are discussed in Chapter 4.

Many people who have CMI also have other unexplained conditions with shared symptoms (such as chronic fatigue syndrome [CFS], fibromyalgia, and irritable bowel syndrome) and may have comorbid conditions (such as depression and anxiety). As summarized in Chapter 5, the committee reviewed treatments for the related and comorbid conditions in an attempt to identify treatments potentially beneficial for people who have CMI. For that review, the committee relied on current evidence-based clinical practice guidelines from government and scientific organizations and existing systematic reviews, rather than conduct a de novo evaluation of the primary literature.

Managing patients who have CMI involves more than administering a therapy. It requires a broader view of treatment. To explore other aspects of care, the committee drew on multiple sources (such as the scientific literature, government reports, care programs used by organizations, and testimony from veterans and their families) so that it could offer recommendations to the Department of Veterans Affairs (VA) aimed at improving its model of care for veterans who have CMI, educating VA clinicians to improve their knowledge on caring for these patients, and improving communication between clinicians and the patients (see Chapters 6 and 7).

SYSTEMATIC REVIEW OF TREATMENTS FOR
CHRONIC MULTISYMPTOM ILLNESS

The committee conducted a systematic review of treatments for CMI, following guidance in *Finding What Works in Health Care: Standards for Systematic Reviews* (IOM, 2011) and the *Cochrane Handbook for Systematic Reviews of Interventions* (Higgins and Green, 2011).

In January 2012, a number of reference databases—PubMed, Embase, The Cochrane Library (Cochrane Central Register of Controlled Trials, Health Technology Assessment, Cochrane Database of Systematic Reviews, Database of Abstracts of Reviews of Effectiveness [DARE]), American College of Physicians (ACP) Journal Club, PsycINFO, and Web of Science— were searched by using terms relevant to treatment for CMI.[1] An additional database, Cumulative Index to Nursing and Allied Health Literature (CINAHL), was searched in April 2012. The search was limited to literature published in 2000–2012 to identify evidence that had become available since a previous Institute of Medicine report, *Gulf War Veterans: Treating Symptoms and Syndromes* (IOM, 2001) was released. Searches were limited to adult populations. Additional potentially eligible studies were identified by hand searching of reference lists of relevant review articles.

Gray-literature sources were searched in April 2012 by using the approach outlined in *Grey Matters: A Practical Search Tool for Evidence-Based Medicine* (CADTH, 2011). Sources searched included the Food and Drug Administration, VA, Health Canada, the Australian Government Department of Health and Aging, the European Commission on Public Health, the System for Information on Grey Literature in Europe, Veterans Affairs Canada, and the Agency for Healthcare Research and Quality (AHRQ). Databases of clinical trials (Congressionally Directed Medical Research Programs, DeployMed ResearchLINK, BioMed Central current controlled trials, International Federation of Pharmaceutical Manufacturers and Associations clinical-trials portal, Thomson CenterWatch Clinical Trials Listing Service, UK Clinical Research Network Study Portfolio, US National Institutes of Health's ClinicalTrials.gov, and World Health Organization International Clinical Trials Registry Platform Search Portal) and clinical practice guidelines (for example, the VA–Department of Defense [VA–DOD] Clinical Practice Guidelines website and the National Guideline Clearing House) were also included in the search. Search terms included *CMI, Gulf War syndrome, Gulf War illness, unexplained illness, undiagnosed illnesses, undiagnosed symptoms, medically unexplained symptoms, somatoform disorder, fatigue, pain, concentration, memory, headaches,* and

---

[1]The strategy used to search PubMed can be found in the public-access file for this study. For information on accessing the public-access file, visit http://www8.nationalacademies.org/ cp/projectview.aspx?key=49452.

gastrointestinal symptoms. In addition to consideration for the systematic review, the search identified relevant resources for use in other parts of the report.

Selection of Evidence

Two reviewers independently screened the search results at the title and abstract level to exclude studies that

- Contained no original data (for example, commentaries and narrative reviews; systematic reviews and meta-analyses were not excluded).
- Described only a case or case series.
- Did not assess medically unexplained symptoms.
- Described only one symptom in the general population (studies of one symptom in military or veteran populations were not excluded).
- Did not describe the results of a treatment or intervention.
- Described only defined syndromes (such as CFS, fibromyalgia, and functional gastrointestinal disorders).
- Did not include humans.
- Did not include an adult population.
- Were published before 2000.

No limits based on study design were used. References that the two reviewers agreed should be excluded were removed from further consideration. References that the two reviewers disagreed about remained for full-text screening. Non-English-language citations were translated, where necessary, to determine eligibility.

After the title and abstract screen, two reviewers independently screened the references remaining by using the full-text articles. In addition to the eligibility criteria applied during the title and abstract screen, they excluded citations at this level that were only meeting abstracts, that were systematic reviews that had been updated, or that described only study protocols but had no results. Disagreements between the reviewers on whether an article should be excluded were resolved by consulting a third reviewer.[2]

Summary of the Literature Search and Study Selection Process

Searches identified 6,541 unique references. After exclusion at the abstract and full-text levels according to the criteria described above,

---

[2]References excluded at the full-text level and the reasons for their exclusion can be found in the public-access file for this study; see http://www8.nationalacademies.org/cp/projectview. aspx?key=49452.

47 studies remained for committee evaluation. Figure 3-1 summarizes the search process.

Data Abstraction and Assessment

Data were abstracted from the eligible studies into tables describing study design, population, intervention, outcomes, and risk of bias. Risk of bias was assessed by using study-design–specific tools: the Cochrane Risk of Bias Tool was used to evaluate controlled trials (Higgins and Green, 2011), and Assessment of Multiple Systematic Reviews (AMSTAR) was used to evaluate systematic reviews (Shea et al., 2007). Studies were grouped by type of intervention, and each group of studies was later evaluated by two committee members.

Chapter 4 summarizes the evidence on each type of intervention. The body of evidence was evaluated for each intervention according to the strength-of-evidence guidance developed by AHRQ (Owens et al., 2010). The AHRQ grading scheme is presented in Table 3-1. To make the determination, the committee examined risk of bias, consistency, directness, and precision of the body of evidence for each intervention.

TREATMENTS FOR COMORBID CONDITIONS WITH SHARED SYMPTOMS

To augment the systematic review of treatments for CMI, the committee also reviewed treatments for other conditions that are closely related to it (see Chapter 5). The committee first identified conditions that are commonly comorbid with CMI or exhibit symptoms that are similar to those seen in people who have CMI. The committee believes that symptoms shared by CMI and the other conditions may respond similarly to approaches to symptom management.

Twelve commonly comorbid conditions or conditions with shared symptoms were identified: fibromyalgia, chronic pain, CFS, somatic symptom disorders, sleep disorders, functional gastrointestinal disorders, depression, anxiety, posttraumatic stress disorder, traumatic brain injury, substance use and addictive disorders, and self-harm. For those conditions, the committee relied on existing systematic reviews and evidence-based clinical practice guidelines to identify the most effective treatment and management techniques. Systematic reviews were collected in March 2012 by searches of several bibliographic databases (PubMed, EMBASE, PsycINFO, Evidence-based Medicine Reviews files in Ovid: Cochrane Database of Systematic Reviews, ACP Journal Club, and DARE). Evidence-based clinical practice guidelines were identified by searches of the National Guideline Clearinghouse, which contains systematically developed evidence-based

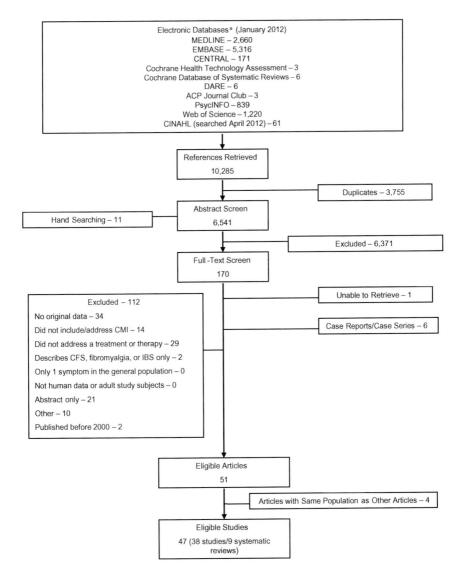

FIGURE 3-1 Summary of search and review process.
[a]MEDLINE accessed via PubMed.
NOTE: ACP = American College of Physicians; CENTRAL = Cochrane Central Register of Controlled Trials; CFS = chronic fatigue syndrome; CINAHL = Cumulative Index to Nursing and Allied Health Literature; DARE = Database of Abstracts of Reviews of Effectiveness; EMBASE = Excerpta Medica database; IBS = irritable bowel syndrome.

TABLE 3-1 AHRQ's Strength-of-Evidence Grades and Definitions

Grade	Definition
High	High confidence that the evidence reflects the true effect. Further research is very unlikely to change the confidence in the estimate of effect.
Moderate	Moderate confidence that the evidence reflects the true effect. Further research may change the confidence in the estimate of effect and may change the estimate.
Low	Low confidence that the evidence reflects the true effect. Further research is likely to change the confidence in the estimate of effect and is likely to change the estimate.
Insufficient	Evidence either is unavailable or does not permit a conclusion.

SOURCE: Reprinted from Owens et al., 2010. Copyright 2010, with permission from Elsevier.

guidelines. Chapter 5 summarizes the existing evidence on conditions that are comorbid and have shared symptoms with CMI.

ADDITIONAL SOURCES OF INFORMATION

As stated above, the committee reviewed several sources of information in addition to the scientific and medical literature to accomplish its task. Three meetings open to the public were held to hear from invited speakers. Presentation topics included general information on CMI, current practices and capabilities in the Veterans Health Administration, current understanding of the underlying mechanism of CMI, treatments for CMI, and how health information technology is being used in managing chronic conditions. Members of the public were given the opportunity to share information and experiences with the committee at the public meetings. Written materials submitted by the public also were considered by the committee.

To understand better the experiences of veterans who have CMI, the committee commissioned an analysis of social media. The analysis, conducted by ConsumerSphere, collected social media discussion data of veterans and their families to describe experiences with CMI in the VA health care system. The program used Web-scraping technology that collects all text, including conversations and discussion, on social media, for example, blogs and microblogs (such as Twitter), message boards, forums, and social networks (such as Facebook). In some cases, Google searches also were conducted. All the information in question is in the public domain. Data were collected for a 12-month period. More than 275,000 conversations, messages, and threads were analyzed. The collected data were analyzed with text analytics programs that used natural-language processing, which allowed an assessment of trends and patterns, connections, and networks; and relevance and associative relationships among the key words. The results, used to inform the committee about veterans' perception of the patient–clinician relationship (Chapter 6) and their satisfaction with VHA care (Chapter 7), are a combination of quantitative and qualitative information.

CURRENT RESEARCH ON CHRONIC MULTISYMPTOM ILLNESS

As part of its information gathering, the committee searched clinical-trial databases (Congressionally Directed Medical Research Programs, DeployMed ResearchLINK, BioMed Central current controlled trials, International Federation of Pharmaceutical Manufacturers and Associations clinical-trials portal, Thomson CenterWatch Clinical Trials Listing Service, UK Clinical Research Network Study Portfolio, US National Institutes of Health's ClinicalTrials.gov, and World Health Organization International Clinical Trials Registry Platform Search Portal) and identified a number of current research projects on CMI treatments. The research is funded largely by VA and DOD. Research projects on CMI treatment deal with, for example, the use of drugs (such as naltrexone, dextromethorphan, and mifepristone), supplements (such as coenzyme Q10 and Sentra), complementary medicine and alternative medicine therapies (such as acupuncture), exercise, mind–body programs, environmental medicine (that is, being in an environment with clear air, eating organic food, and drinking filtered water), and telemedicine. Other research projects are studying the mechanisms of CMI. Because the current research has not yet been completed or results were not available in the published literature, the committee was not able to evaluate it for inclusion in the present report.

REFERENCES

CADTH (Canadian Agency for Drugs and Technologies in Health). 2011. *Grey Matters: A Practical Search Tool for Evidence-Based Medicine.*

Higgins, J. P. T., and S. Green, eds. 2011. *Cochrane Handbook for Systematic Reviews of Interventions.* Version 5.1.0: The Cochrane Collaboration.

IOM (Institute of Medicine). 2001. *Gulf War Veterans: Treating Symptoms and Syndromes, The Compass Series.* Washington, DC: National Academy Press.

IOM. 2011. *Finding What Works in Health Care: Standards for Systematic Reviews.* Washington, DC: The National Academies Press.

Owens, D. K., K. N. Lohr, D. Atkins, J. R. Treadwell, J. T. Reston, E. B. Bass, S. Chang, and M. Helfand. 2010. AHRQ series paper 5: Grading the strength of a body of evidence when comparing medical interventions: Agency for Healthcare Research and Quality and the Effective Health-Care Program. *Journal of Clinical Epidemiology* 63(5):513-523.

Shea, B. J., J. M. Grimshaw, G. A. Wells, M. Boers, N. Andersson, C. Hamel, A. C. Porter, P. Tugwell, D. Moher, and L. M. Bouter. 2007. Development of AMSTAR: A measurement tool to assess the methodological quality of systematic reviews. *BMC Medical Research Methodology* 7(10): doi:10.1186/1471-2288-7-10.

4

Treatment for
Chronic Multisymptom Illness

This chapter assesses the evidence on interventions for treatment for symptoms associated with, or that define, chronic multisymptom illness (CMI). The 38 studies and nine systematic reviews (described in 51 manuscripts) reviewed were found in the systematic search detailed in Chapter 3 for treatments of multiple physical symptoms associated with CMI. A narrative synthesis of the evidence is presented here by type of treatment: pharmacologic treatments and other biologic interventions, psychotherapies, mind–body approaches (including biofeedback, cognitive rehabilitation therapy, and complementary and alternative therapies), and exercise interventions. The committee looked for evidence of efficacy or effectiveness[1] of interventions in alleviating symptoms and improving quality of life in all populations affected by multiple symptoms or syndromes similar to CMI. This chapter also includes the committee's evaluation of the body of evidence on each treatment on the basis of the Agency for Healthcare Research and Quality (AHRQ) strength-of-evidence grading (Owens et al., 2010) and conclusions about the effectiveness of the evaluated treatments.

The committee did not limit its investigation to particular types of treatments but rather chose to evaluate all treatments on which there was evidence. The treatments considered varied widely and included nontraditional medicine, such as complementary and alternative medicine,

---

[1]Efficacy is benefit from an intervention under the best possible conditions, such as in a randomized controlled trial in which a selected sample of a specific population is carefully monitored by physicians, whereas effectiveness is benefit in real life as shown by many types of research studies (Agency for Healthcare Research and Quality, 2011).

psychologic therapies, and stress-management techniques. The committee also considered various outcomes, including symptoms, functioning, quality of life, health care use, and harms. Although the symptoms of CMI are physical, the committee embraced the need for a "whole-person" approach because of the complexity of CMI and its potential comorbidities. The nontraditional treatments were included in an effort to identify potentially effective pathways for treatment of the whole person instead of focusing on each specific symptom.

Only three studies that were identified were conducted in samples of veterans. Each reported the effects of a different intervention: cognitive rehabilitation therapy (Jakcsy, 2002), doxycycline (Donta et al., 2004), and cognitive behavioral therapy (CBT) and exercise (Donta et al., 2003; Guarino et al., 2001; Mori et al., 2006). The veteran populations were generally male (85% in Donta et al., 2003, and Mori et al., 2006; 86% in Donta et al., 2004, and 50% in Jakcsy, 2002), and the average age ranged from 37.5 years (Jakcsy, 2002) to 40.7 years (Donta et al., 2004). The committee considers those studies with others of similar interventions but different populations below.

The committee believed it necessary to consider additional evidence so that it could offer recommendations about the best treatment and management approaches for veterans who have CMI. Thus, the recommendations presented in Chapter 8 result from careful consideration of the evidence presented in the present chapter, evidence on the best treatments for comorbid and related conditions in Chapter 5, and issues surrounding patient care and communication in Chapters 6 and 7.

PHARMACOLOGIC INTERVENTIONS

People who have many of the conditions described in this report are treated with pharmacologic agents that are also used to treat for other conditions. Often, the mechanisms of action of the pharmacologic agents are unknown. For example, patients who have fibromyalgia may benefit from duloxetine, which works independently of depression (which duloxetine is often prescribed for). Such agents include selective serotonin reuptake inhibitors, serotonin–norepinephrine reuptake inhibitors (for example, duloxetine), tricyclic medications (for example, amitriptyline), monoamine oxidase inhibitors (for example, phenelzine), dopaminergic blockers (for example, haloperidol), anxiolytics (for example, benzodiazepines), and medications that potentiate gaba-ergic transmission (for example, gabapentin), potentiate binding of voltage-gated calcium channels (for example, pregabalin), and potentiate voltage-dependent sodium channels (for example, topiramate). Analgesic medications include nonsteroidal anti-inflammatory analgesics, acetaminophen, opioid analgesics, and tramadol, which is serotonergic and partially binds to the mu-opiate receptor. Because of the variety of effects of these pharmacologic agents and their varied biologic targets, the committee considered the evidence on specific agents rather than broad classes.

The committee reviewed 11 studies: nine clinical studies and two systematic reviews. Of the clinical trials, five were randomized (Donta et al., 2004; Han et al., 2008a; Kroenke et al., 2006; Muller et al., 2008; Volz et al., 2000), six were blinded (Altamura et al., 2003; Donta et al., 2004; Han et al., 2008a; Kroenke et al., 2006; Muller et al., 2008; Volz et al., 2000), and three were pre–post[2] studies (Garcia-Campayo and Sanz-Carrillo, 2002; Han et al., 2008b; Menza et al., 2001). Six of the clinical trials included agents typically known as antidepressants (mirtazapine, venlafaxine, nefazodone, escitalopram, paroxetine, and opipramol), one an antipsychotic (sulpiride), one an anticonvulsant (topiramate), and one an antibiotic (doxycycline).

Most of the pharmacologic studies were limited by a high number of dropouts in both treatment and placebo arms. Only one study involved the veteran population (Donta et al., 2004); it was the only study that used a nonpsychopharmacologic intervention (doxycycline), and it did not demonstrate efficacy. The other eight studies enrolled people in the general population, most of them female, who had somatoform disorder variously described as multisomatoform disorder, undifferentiated somatoform disorder, and somatization disorder. Two studies excluded patients who had comorbid major depressive disorder, social anxiety disorder, or generalized anxiety disorder but used anxiolytics, alprazolam, or lorazepam in over 50% of the subjects in addition to the medications being assessed (Han et al., 2008a,b). The generalizability of studies of nonveteran populations to the veteran population is unclear.

In all the studies except the doxycycline study (Donta et al., 2004), the authors concluded that there may be benefit from specific drug interventions but that future research should include larger cohorts of patients and fixed doses of medications. The evidence is limited by small sample sizes, high dropout rates, and potentially confounding effects of depression and anxiety. The influence of pharmaceutical manufacturers, who funded or employed the authors of several of the clinical trials, may have affected the reported results (Altamura et al., 2003; Donta et al., 2004; Han et al., 2008a; Kroenke et al., 2006; Menza et al., 2001). Publication bias may also be an issue if it limited the evidence available for consideration by the committee.

Regarding the risk of bias in each study, the committee judged four of the studies (Donta et al., 2004; Kroenke et al., 2006; Muller et al., 2008;

---

[2]Pre–post is used to describe clinical study designs where pre-intervention measures are compared to post-intervention measures.

Volz et al., 2000) to be at low risk for bias and five to be at high risk (Altamura et al., 2003; Garcia-Campayo and Sanz-Carrillo, 2002; Han et al., 2008a,b; Menza et al., 2001).

The two systematic reviews were of relatively good quality. A review by Sumathipala et al. (2007) was particularly relevant in that the studies reviewed focused on adults who had medically unexplained symptoms and excluded symptom syndromes such as chronic fatigue syndrome (CFS), fibromyalgia, and irritable bowel syndrome (IBS). The studies that were reviewed were limited by high dropout rates, focus on short-term outcomes, and use of varied methods but did indicate support for antidepressants. A review by Kroenke (2007) noted that pharmacologic studies were limited by short follow-up and included drugs that are not available in the United States.

On the basis of guidance provided by AHRQ (Owens et al., 2010), the committee rated the strength of evidence as shown in Table 4-1 and concluded that

- There is *insufficient* strength of evidence to determine the effectiveness of paroxetine, nefazodone, and opipramol in people who have somatoform disorders.
- There is *low* strength of evidence that venlafaxine, escitalopram, levosulpiride, and topiramate improved symptoms in people who had somatoform disorders.
- There is *high* strength of evidence that doxycycline is *not* effective in improving symptoms and functioning in veterans who have CMI (referred to as Gulf War illnesses in Donta et al., 2004).

Each of the studies on pharmacologic interventions is summarized in Table 4-2. Clinical trials are presented first, followed by systematic reviews.

OTHER BIOLOGIC INTERVENTIONS

Fontani et al. (2011) studied the use of noninvasive radioelectric asymmetric conveyer brain stimulation (REAC-BS) to treat for pain and physical problems related to stress. REAC-BS is a series of painless electric pulses applied to specific reflex auricular points. The authors found that patients treated with REAC-BS reported fewer pain and physical symptoms after treatment after a 4-week treatment cycle than those treated with a placebo. The study was limited because there was a lack of follow-up and because the dose was not standardized but varied on the basis of patient response. Patients may have been able to sense the stimulations and deduce their allocation to the treatment or placebo group. The clinical significance of pre–post score change from 122 to 96 on the psychologic stress measure questionnaire is unclear (Fontani et al., 2011).

TABLE 4-1 Strength of Evidence on Pharmacologic Interventions

No. Studies (No. Subjects)	RoB	Consistency	Directness	Precision	Strength of Evidence
Venlafaxine					
RCT: 2 (207)[a]	High	Consistent	Indirect	Imprecise	Low
Paroxetine					
Pre–post: 1 (22)[b]	High	N/A	Indirect	Imprecise	Insufficient
Nefazodone					
Pre–post: 1 (15)[c]	High	N/A	Indirect	Imprecise	Insufficient
Escitalopram					
RCT: 1 (31)[d]	Low	N/A	Indirect	Imprecise	Low
Opipramol					
RCT: 1 (208)[e]	Unclear	N/A	Indirect	Imprecise	Insufficient
Levosulpiride					
RCT: 1 (74)[f]	High	N/A	Indirect	Imprecise	Low
Topiramate					
Pre–post: 1 (35)[g]	High	N/A	Direct	Imprecise	Low
Doxycycline					
RCT: 1 (491)[h]	Low	N/A	Direct	Precise	High[i]

NOTES: RCT = randomized controlled trial; RoB = risk of bias.
[a]Han et al., 2008a; Kroenke et al., 2006.
[b]Han et al., 2008b.
[c]Menza et al., 2001.
[d]Muller et al., 2008.
[e]Volz et al., 2000.
[f]Altamura et al., 2003.
[g]Garcia-Campayo and Sanz-Carrillo, 2002.
[h]Donta et al., 2004.
[i]No beneficial effect was found in the study.

On the basis of guidance provided by AHRQ (Owens et al., 2010), the committee rated the strength of evidence as shown in Table 4-3 and found that there was *insufficient* evidence to draw conclusions about the effectiveness of REAC-BS in treating for CMI. Details of Fontani et al. (2011) are summarized in Table 4-4.

PSYCHOTHERAPIES

Cognitive Behavioral Interventions

The committee reviewed five individual CBT studies and five group CBT studies that assessed CBT for patients who presented with somatic symptoms. Somatic-focused CBT, reviewed below, is not general CBT but rather targets somatic symptoms directly and includes relaxation and activity components.

TABLE 4-2 Pharmacologic Interventions

Study	Type	Intervention	Population
Altamura et al., 2003 Somatoform disorders Italy	RCT, crossover	Levosulpiride 50 mg/ day vs placebo for 4 weeks.	64.9% female, mean age 38.1 years N levosulpiride = 37 N placebo = 37
Donta et al., 2004 Veterans with Gulf War veterans illness and positive for mycoplasma DNA US VA and DOD medical centers	RCT	Doxycycline 200 mg/ day vs identically matched placebo capsules for 12 months.	14% female, mean age 41 years N screened = 2,712 N doxycycline = 245 N placebo = 246
Garcia-Campayo and Sanz-Carrillo, 2002 Multisomatoform disorder Zargoza, Spain	Pre–post	Topiramate starting at 50 mg, increased by 50 mg every 4 days to a maximum of 300–400 mg (150–200 mg bi-daily) or until adverse event occurred; trial lasted 6 months; dose averaged 365.7 mg (range 300–400 mg).	68.6% female, mean age 41.8 years N screened = 84 N enrolled = 35
Han et al., 2008a Undifferentiated somatoform disorder Ansan, Korea	RCT	Venlafaxine vs mirtazapine. Venlafaxine starting at 37.5 mg/day, increased each week by 37.5–75 mg/day to maximum of 225 mg/day. Mirtazapine starting at 15 mg/day, increased by 15 mg/ day to maximum of 60 mg/day. Both were adjusted for tolerability and clinical response. Conducted over 12 weeks.	61% female, mean age 45 years N venlafaxine = 45 N mirtazapine = 50

Outcomes and Results

After treatment, levosulpiride patients reported fewer symptoms (measured by CISSD-SDS) compared with baseline (1,709 vs 1,205 symptoms, p = 0.007) and compared with placebo at 4 weeks (1,205 vs 1,597 symptoms, p < 0.001).

No difference between treatments in anticholinergic or neuroendocrine side effects reported; extrapyramidal system involvement was reported more frequently by levosulpiride-treated patients (9 vs 2 patients, p < 0.03).

After treatment, treatment and placebo groups did not differ significantly in any outcome measured. In primary outcome, physical health functioning (SF-36), treatment and placebo groups' average scores were 30.2 and 30.1 (physical) and 37.4 and 36.2 (mental), respectively, at baseline; at 12 months, treatment and placebo groups' average scores were 32.0 and 30.9 (physical) and 37.6 and 36.7 (mental). No differences in pain (MPQ), fatigue (MFI), or cognition (Cognitive Failures Questionnaire). After 12 months, 154 of 200 doxycycline and 159 of 211 placebo patients were negative for mycoplasma DNA.

Increased adverse events considered related to study drug were myalgia in placebo group (4.5% vs 1.2%, p = 0.05), nausea in doxycycline group (37.1% vs 10.2%, p < 0.001), and photosensitivity in doxycycline group (14.7% vs 6.1%, p = 0.002); all other reported events were in the two groups.

Blood doxycycline concentrations were undetectable in 38.9% of treatment-group patients and 98% of placebo-group patients at 12 months (adherence).

From baseline to 6-month follow-up, improvements in severity (CGI, 3.8 to 3.3, p < 0.001) and functioning (GAF, 52.4 to 58.5, p < 0.001) were significant; no significant changes were seen in pain (pain VAS, 68.8 to 68.7; MPQ, 36.6 to 36.2) or anxiety and depression (HADS, 9.5 to 9.6).

Most frequently reported side effects were somnolence (25.7%), fatigue (20%), paresthesia (14.2%), nervousness (8.5%), and nausea (5.7%).

After treatment, mean somatic symptom severity scores (PHQ-15) decreased significantly for mirtazapine (–8.4, p < 0.0001) and venlafaxine (–6.1, p < 0.0001) over 12 weeks; between-group difference was significant (p = 0.046) in favor of mirtazapine.

For mirtazapine, scores for psychologic distress (GHQ-12) and depression (BDI) decreased significantly between baseline and end of study (–4.9, p < 0.0001 and –13.5, p < 0.0001, respectively); for venlafaxine, psychologic distress and depression scores also decreased significantly (–4.3, p = 0.001 and –9.02, p < 0.0001) with no significant difference between groups.

Adverse effects reported by participants were dry mouth in both groups; somnolence, yawning, and dizziness in mirtazapine group; and nausea in venlafaxine group.

continued

TABLE 4-2 Continued

Study	Type	Intervention	Population
Han et al., 2008b Undifferentiated somatoform disorder Ansan, Korea	Pre–post	Paroxetine Immediate Release (IR) administered starting at 10 mg/day and increased to a maximum of 40 mg/day on basis of patient's response over 8 weeks; average dose was 19.5 mg/day (range 10–40 mg/day).	59% female, mean age 37.4 years N screened = 43 N enrolled = 22
Kroenke et al., 2006 Multisomatoform disorder USA	RCT	Venlafaxine ER vs placebo. Capsules given once a day in following doses: week 1 = 75 mg; week 2 = 150 mg; weeks 3–12 = 225 mg. Dose was decreased to tolerable level for participants who experienced intolerance. Conducted over 12 weeks, with up to 2 weeks of taper.	80% female, mean age 47 years N screened = 231 N venlafaxine ER = 55 N placebo = 57
Menza et al., 2001 Somatization disorder Piscataway, New Jersey	Pre–post	Nefazodone administered starting at 50 mg bi-daily, increased to 100 mg bi-daily after first week, increased to 150 mg bi-daily in weeks 2–8.	86% female, mean age 48.6 years N screened = 46 N enrolled = 15

Outcomes and Results

After treatment, average symptom severity (PHQ-15) score dropped significantly, by 75%, from 17.2 to 4.3 (p = 0.001) between baseline and 8 weeks. Average depression (BDI) scores also decreased significantly, 50.8% (p < 0.001), and average psychologic distress (GHQ-12) scores decreased by 13%, but difference was not significant.
Most common adverse events reported were nausea, dry mouth, and somnolence.

After treatment, both treatment and placebo groups had significant (p < 0.0001) decrease in somatic symptoms (PHQ-15 change of –8.3 and –6.6 respectively) but no significant difference between groups (p = 0.097). From baseline to 12 weeks, greater improvement was seen in Venlafaxine ER participants than in those who received placebo for pain (PHQ-15 pain subscale, –3.3 and –2.6, respectively, p = 0.03), psychic anxiety (HAM-A, –8.6 and –5.9, respectively, p = 0.02), clinical improvement (CGI-Improvement, –1.8 and –1.4, respectively, p = 0.009), physical symptoms (MQOL Physical symptoms, –11.7 and –6.0, respectively, p = 0.01), mental health (SF-36, 28.6 and 16.8, respectively, p = 0.03), bodily pain (SF-36, 26.1 and 14.5, respectively, p = 0.03), and concentration (MOS-CS, 30.1 and 15.3, respectively, p = 0.007).
Significant (p ≤ 0.001) improvement from baseline to week 12 was noted for several measures without difference between groups (depression, HAM-D; HAM-A total score and HAM-A somatic anxiety score; CGI-Severity score; and SF-36 physical health score).
Percentage of patients reporting bothersome headache and stomach pain symptoms decreased significantly more in venlafaxine ER than in placebo-treated patients (both p = 0.03).
Venlafaxine ER–treated participants reported more adverse effects than placebo; more than 10% of venlafaxine ER patients reported nausea, headache, fatigue, dizziness, constipation, and tremor.

11 of 15 patients who completed study showed nonsignificant improvement by 24% in symptom severity on VAS after 8 weeks of treatment compared with baseline. From baseline to week 8, 73% of participants showed improvement on CGI (significance not noted), and 73% showed significant improvement in functioning (SF-36, p < 0.025). Significant improvement in depression (p < 0.005) and cognitive and somatic subscales (both p < 0.025) of HAM-D and HAM-A were reported, but there was no correlation with VAS, CGI, or SF-36 score.
Most common adverse effects were sedation, GI discomfort, anxiety, and dry mouth.

continued

TABLE 4-2 Continued

Study	Type	Intervention	Population
Muller et al., 2008 Multisomatoform disorder Cape Town, South Africa	RCT	Escitalopram vs placebo. Administered at 10 mg/day and could be increased to 20 mg/day after week 4 (dose decreased to 10 mg/day for intolerance). Dosage was constant for weeks 8–12; after 12 weeks, dosage was tapered and stopped over 1 week. Entire study took place over 18 months.	90% female, mean age 40 years N screened = 60 N escitalopram = 25 N placebo = 26
Volz et al., 2000 Somatoform disorders (ICD-10 codes F45.0, F45.1, F45.3) Germany	RCT	Opipramol vs placebo. Started at 50 mg/day, increased by 50–200 mg/day on day 4. Number of placebo capsules was identical with number of opipramol capsules. Treatment lasted 6 weeks.	64% female, mean age 46 years N opipramol = 104 N placebo = 104
Systematic Reviews			
Kroenke, 2007 Somatoform disorders	Systematic review	Multiple	N RCTs = 34
Sumathipala, 2007 Somatoform disorders	Systematic review	Multiple	N abstracts screened = 368 N systematic reviews = 6 N RCTs = 14

Outcomes and Results

After treatment, symptom severity (PHQ-15) scores in treatment group decreased significantly more than in placebo group (14.6 vs 17.3 at baseline and 5.6 vs 12.5 at 12 weeks, respectively, p < 0.0001). Clinical improvement (CGI-Improvement, treatment: 3.0 to 1.6 vs placebo: 3.4 to 3.2, at baseline and 12 weeks, respectively) and severity (CGI-Severity, treatment: 4.5 to 2.6 vs placebo: 4.7 to 4.1, at baseline and 12 weeks, respectively) also showed significant improvement in treatment subjects (p < 0.05).

Likewise, escitalopram showed improvement on somatic anxiety (HAM-A somatic subscore, p < 0.0001, and HAM-A psychic subscore, p = 0.0002), depression (MADRS, p = 0.017), and disability (SDS, p = 0.015) scores after 12 weeks compared with placebo. No difference between treatment and placebo in illness behavior (SAIB) was detected.

After 12 weeks, 80% of treatment and 26.9% of placebo subjects met criteria for being responsive to treatment, and 52% of treatment and 3.8% of placebo subjects met criteria for remission.

Most common adverse events were headache, nausea, and abdominal discomfort in first 2 weeks and headache, nasopharyngitis, and diarrhea in weeks 2–12, with no significant differences between treatment and placebo groups in reported adverse events.

Average dose was 14.4 mg of escitalopram per day and 18.1 mg of placebo per day.

After treatment, anxiety scores decreased significantly more in opipramol group than in placebo group for somatic anxiety (HAM-A somatic subscore, 16.8 to 7.3 vs 16.9 to 9.1, p = 0.013) and total anxiety (HAM-A, 25.1 to 11.8 vs 25.3 to 14.5, p = 0.013), and decrease in psychic anxiety score was nearly significant (HAM-A psychic subscore, 8.3 to 4.5 vs 8.4 to 5.4, p = 0.052). Scores followed same trend with greater decrease in opipramol group and in placebo group for depression (HAM-D, 14.6 to 8.0 vs 14.3 to 9.5, p = 0.006) and for symptoms (SCLR-90-R, 0.95 to 0.57 vs 0.77 to 0.55, p = 0.041), including somatic symptoms (1.61 to 0.93 vs 1.40 to 0.98, p = 0.043) and anxiety symptoms (1.15 to 0.63 vs 0.94 to 0.64, p = 0.049).

Adverse events were reported by 37% of opipramol patients and 38% of placebo patients—gastrointestinal complaints in 7.1% of opipramol patients and 20.8% of placebo patients and musculoskeletal complaints in 14% of opipramol patients and 7% of placebo patients. Tiredness occurred more frequently in opipramol group than in placebo group (9% vs 2%).

Positive results for at least one outcome (symptoms, functional, or psychologic) were noted in 11 of 13 CBT studies and 4 of 5 antidepressants studies, and 8 of 16 studies of other interventions reported improvement—consultation letter to primary care physician (4 studies), primary care physician training (2 studies), and non-CBT psychotherapies (2 studies), hypnosis (2 studies), and one study each investigating multicomponent nurse-care management, aerobic exercise, writing disclosure, paradoxic intention, and explanatory therapy.

CBT is most effective for variety of somatoform disorders and outcomes.

Studies assessed interventions with antidepressants (1 review and 3 RCTs), CBT (5 reviews and 2 RCTs), psychiatric consultation (3 RCTs), other forms of psychotherapy (3 RCTs), exercise (2 RCTs), and collaborative care (1 RCT).

Studies have many limitations and varied methods, so interventions cannot be compared. Authors note support for antidepressants and CBT and limited evidence on other interventions.

continued

TABLE 4-2 Continued

NOTES: BDI = Beck Depression Inventory; CGI = Clinical Global Impressions Scale; CISSD-SDS = Conceptual Issues in Somatoform and Similar Disorders, somatoform disorders schedule; GAF = Global Assessment of Functioning; GHQ-12 = 12-item General Health Questionnaire; HADS = Hospital Anxiety and Depression Scale; HAM-A = Hamilton Anxiety Rating Scale; HAM-D = Hamilton Depression Rating Scale; MADRS = Montgomery–Åsberg Depression Rating Scale; MFI = Multidimensional Fatigue Inventory; MPQ = McGill Pain Questionnaire; MQOL = McGill Quality of Life Questionnaire; MOS-CS = Medical Outcomes Study Concentration Scale; PHQ-15 = Patient Health Questionnaire 15-Item Somatic Symptom Severity Scale; RCT = randomized controlled trial; SAIB = Scale for the Assessment of Illness Behaviour; SCL-90-R = Symptom Checklist-90-Revised; SDS = Sheehan Disability Scale; SF-36 = Medical Outcomes Study 36-Item Short Form Health Survey; VAS = Visual Analogue Scale.

TABLE 4-3 Strength of Evidence on Other Biologic Interventions

No. Studies (No. Subjects)	RoB	Consistency	Directness	Precision	Strength of Evidence
REAC-BS RCT: 1 (888)[a]	Low	N/A	Indirect	Precise	Insufficient

NOTES: RCT = randomized controlled trial; REAC-BS = radioelectric asymmetric conveyer brain stimulation; RoB = risk of bias.
[a]Fontani et al., 2011.

TABLE 4-4 Other Biologic Interventions

Study	Type	Intervention	Size
Fontani et al., 2011 Pain and physical problems and medically unexplained symptoms Florence, Italy	RCT	Noninvasive REAC-BS or inactive REAC: 18 sessions of 7 pulses on alternating days over 4 weeks.	77% female, mean age 43 years N REAC = 688 N inactive REAC = 200

NOTE: PSM = Psychological Stress Measure; RCT = randomized controlled trial; REAC-BS = radioelectric asymmetric conveyer brain stimulation; SD = standard deviation.

In general, the goals of somatic-focused CBT are to modify dysfunctional beliefs about symptoms, reduce psychophysiologic arousal through relaxation, enhance activity regulation through increased exercise and pleasurable activities, and increase awareness and enhance communication of thoughts and emotions. Therapy is usually brief, ranging from 5 to 12 weekly therapy sessions.

Individual Cognitive Behavioral Interventions

Of the six clinical trials of individual sessions, all but one (Arnold et al., 2009) were RCTs (Allen et al., 2006; Escobar et al., 2007; Sharpe et al., 2011; Sumathipala et al., 2000, 2008). CBT in those trials ranged from 5 to 12 individual sessions, typically administered weekly for about 50–90 minutes in a mental health specialty clinic or a primary care (PC) clinic, most often by a mental health professional but some by a PC physician. Components of the CBT included various behavioral and cognitive techniques, including time-contingent activity planning, pleasant-activity scheduling, sleep hygiene, cognitive restructuring of negative thinking, affect management, and problem-solving skills. Most trials used standard medical care, routine clinical care, psychiatric consultation, or treatment as usual as the control condition. In two instances, a consultation letter to the PC physician was added to the control condition (Allen et al., 2006; Escobar et al., 2007). Most of the studies targeted somatoform conditions, including mainly somatization disorder, abridged somatization, and high levels of unexplained physical symptoms. Moreover, substantial comorbidity, particularly anxiety and depressive syndromes, was documented in the studies.

All the RCTs reported at least some benefit from the intervention (Allen et al., 2006; Escobar et al., 2007; Sharpe et al., 2011; Sumathipala et al., 2000, 2008). Most of the studies documented a consistent, beneficial effect

---

Outcomes and Results

At baseline, average total pain and physical problems (PSM) score was 122.53 (SD ± 6.75) in treatment group and 122.96 (SD ± 7.04) in placebo group. After treatment, average total scores for treatment and placebo groups were 96.01 (SD ± 8.5) and 122.11 (SD ± 7.5), respectively, with significant decrease in PSM score in treated subjects ($p < 0.005$) but no change in placebo group. In number-needed-to-treat analysis, there were 403 of 688 subjects positive for stress-related pain and physical problems in treatment group and 159 of 200 in placebo group; after treatment, 196 of 403 (48.6%, asymptotic significance = 0.000) in treatment group and 135 of 158 (84.9%) in placebo group remained positive for stress-related pain and physical problems.
RR = 0.42; number needed to treat = 2.56.

of CBT relative to the control condition, most notably immediately after treatment, with gains largely maintained through long-term follow-up, which was up to 15 months (Allen et al., 2006). The pattern of improvement was largely consistent in all assessed outcomes, including assessment of physical symptoms by a blind interviewer and self-reported physical symptoms, such psychiatric symptoms as depression and anxiety, patient satisfaction, and measures of functioning. Retention rates were generally similar in the CBT and control groups (about 10–30%) and appear to compare favorably with rates for other interventions (such as medications) and with rates in the broader CBT literature for such mental disorders as depression and posttraumatic stress disorder. Generally, sample sizes in the RCTs were appropriate for detecting large, clinically significant effects.

Four of the individual studies (Allen et al., 2006; Escobar et al., 2007; Sharpe et al., 2011; Sumathipala et al., 2000, 2008) can be viewed as predominantly low risk of bias and one as high risk (Arnold et al., 2009).

Group Cognitive Behavioral Interventions

Five studies examined group CBT (Bleichhardt et al., 2004; Donta et al., 2003; Lidbeck, 2003; Martin et al., 2007; Mori et al., 2006; Rief et al., 2002; Zaby et al., 2008). The Lidbeck (2003) study included patients who met criteria for functional somatic symptoms, including hypochondriasis and irritable colon syndrome. The study by Bleichhardt et al. (2004) and Rief et al. (2002) and that by Zaby et al. (2008) examined multiple somatoform symptoms. Finally, the study by Donta et al. (2003) and Martin et al. (2007) examined medically unexplained symptoms. Interventions were conducted in a one- to eight-session group format with groups of up to 10. Interventions were typically carried out in a PC setting or a specialized setting with a trained psychotherapist. Only one of the studies was conducted in military or veteran samples (Donta et al., 2003; Mori et al., 2006).

Of the cognitive behavioral group interventions, four (Bleichhardt et al., 2004; Donta et al., 2003; Martin et al., 2007; Mori et al., 2006; Rief et al., 2002; Zaby et al., 2008) were original studies, and one was a follow-up of an earlier clinical trial (Lidbeck, 2003). The largest study, in which 1,092 Gulf War veterans who had multisymptom illness were enrolled, compared CBT plus exercise, CBT alone, exercise alone, and usual care (Donta et al., 2003; Guarino et al., 2001; Mori et al., 2006). For the main outcome of physical functioning, the group receiving CBT had an odds ratio (OR) of 1.73 (95% confidence interval [CI] 1.21–2.41) compared with no CBT, and exercise had an OR of 1.00 (95% CI 0.76–1.50) compared with no exercise. Those results suggest that group CBT rather than exercise conferred the main therapeutic benefit with respect to physical symptoms. Adherence (attendance to 8 out of 12 CBT or exercise sessions) was not related to changes in physical function in the CBT group; however, adherent exercise participants were twice as likely than nonadherent participants to improve (p = 0.02). In a secondary data analysis, however, exercise alone or in combination with group CBT showed improvement in fatigue (general, physical, mental, activity level, and motivation). The observed sizes of treatment effects were lower than reported in other trials, and this might reflect the group format of CBT, the low number of sessions attended (6 of 12 exercise sessions or 5 of 12 CBT sessions attended on average), the range of therapist experience, and variability in the administration of CBT among sites.

Bleichhardt et al. (2004) and Rief et al. (2002) examined standard treatment plus either a specific somatic intervention or relaxation (another CBT intervention), and a waitlist control (N = 191). In the analyses, only the randomized arms for somatic-specific CBT intervention and relaxation were examined, and they showed small to large treatment effects through 1-year follow-up, with the largest effects on reduction in number of somatoform symptoms. There were no differences between the somatic CBT and relaxation groups except the lower number of doctor visits in the somatic CBT group. In the waitlist control group, there were no changes over the 4-month waiting period.

Martin et al. (2007) examined patients who had medically unexplained symptoms (N = 140), comparing one session of 3–4 hours of group CBT with standard medical care. Through a 6-month follow-up, patients in both groups showed improvements; there was greater reduction in doctor visits and somatization severity after CBT than after standard care.

In a study similar to that of Bleichhardt et al. (2004), Zaby et al. (2008), in a smaller sample (N = 77), showed a moderate decrease in somatic symptoms after both a specific somatic CBT therapy and relaxation and little improvement in a separate waitlist condition. The specific CBT somatic therapy also reduced anxiety and improved mental health compared with relaxation. Relaxation in both studies consisted of progressive muscle relaxation. Lidbeck et al. (2003), in a smaller follow-up (N = 31) of an RCT (Lidbeck, 1997), showed sustained improvement at 6-month follow-up after CBT somatic intervention.

The committee found that the studies of group CBT were of low risk of bias.

Brief Psychodynamic Psychotherapy Interventions

The committee reviewed four individual clinical studies and one study of group intervention published after 2000 that have examined brief psychodynamic psychologic interventions (typically fewer than 12 sessions).

Individual Psychodynamic Psychotherapies

Five of the studies examined brief individual dynamic or brief psycho-dynamic therapies in people who had medically unexplained symptoms (Abbass et al., 2009a; Aiarzaguena et al., 2002), multisomatoform disorder (Sattel et al., 2012), functional neurologic symptoms (Reuber et al., 2007), and alexithymia with somatization (Posse, 2004). Reuber et al. (2007) and Posse (2004) included too little information for determining how similar or dissimilar the diagnosis was to CMI. There were problems related to stan-dardization of therapy—such as a lack of a detailed therapy manual (Abbass et al., 2009a; Aiarzaguena et al., 2002; Posse, 2004; Reuber et al., 2007), the use of only one therapist (Posse, 2004; Reuber et al., 2007), failure to assess therapeutic adherence (Aiarzaguena et al., 2002; Posse, 2004; Reuber et al., 2007), or lack of acceptable therapeutic adherence (Sattel et al., 2012). Both Reuber et al. (2007) and Sattel et al. (2012) noted that components of cogni-tive behavioral approaches were allowed to be included in the intervention. No studies examined military or veteran samples.

Of the individual studies, two (Posse, 2004; Sattel et al., 2012) were RCTs, and three were pre–post designs (Abbass et al., 2009a; Aiarzaguena et al., 2002; Reuber et al., 2007). The Sattel et al. (2012) trial was the largest of the psychodynamic intervention trials, with 211 participants. It compared the results of 12 weekly 90-minute sessions of psychodynamic interpersonal therapy (PIT), including some cognitive behavioral compo-nents, with the results of three 30-minute sessions of enhanced medical care (EMC) separated by about 6 weeks. After treatment, PIT was not superior to EMC on any of the somatic or mental health outcomes. At 9-month follow-up, PIT emerged as superior to EMC only for somatic outcomes, with a small to moderate effect size ($d = 0.42$), but not for mental health or health care use outcomes.

Posse (2004), published in Spanish, reported that five patients who were receiving Jungian therapy improved significantly more than five con-trols on measures of anxiety, fatigue, and impulsivity. However, the study lacked description of methods—including selection and randomization of participants, the intervention, and the control condition—and therefore carries a high risk of bias.

The three brief uncontrolled trials (Abbass et al., 2009a; Aiarzaguena et al., 2002; Reuber et al., 2007) found moderate effects of therapy on out-comes. Abbass et al. (2009a), using open-ended dynamic intervention of one to 25 sessions with 50 participants, showed a 69% reduction ($p < 0.001$) in emergency department visits per person and improved somatic symp-toms. Aiarzaguena et al. (2002), in a small sample of 12 participants with a pre–post structured psychotherapy approach handled by PC physicians, reported improvement in functioning and quality of life. Reuber et al. (2007)

used up to 19 sessions of psychodynamic intervention and failed to show an improvement in intent-to-treat analyses of somatic symptoms in 91 participants but found improvement in general clinical outcome and quality of life.

Of the individual psychodynamic psychotherapy clinical studies, one study (Sattel et al., 2012) was rated as of low risk of bias and the remainder (Abbass et al., 2009a; Aiarzaguena et al., 2002; Reuber et al., 2007) as of high risk of bias.

Group Psychodynamic Psychotherapies

One study used a group intervention based on psychodynamic principles in a sample of people who met criteria for somatoform disorder (Rembold, 2011). This small study (N = 40) reported improvements in number of somatic symptoms, impairment due to symptoms, and anxiety relative to treatment as usual under PC physician control. Although it was promising, lack of reporting of randomization procedures and inferential statistics limits any conclusions that can be drawn from the study. It was rated as of high risk of bias.

Psychotherapy Intervention Reviews

The committee looked at five systematic reviews published after 2000 that examined trials of CBT for patients who presented with somatic symptoms (Kroenke, 2007; Kroenke and Swindle, 2000; Looper and Kirmayer, 2002; Nezu et al., 2001; Sumathipala, 2007), and two meta-analyses (Abbass et al., 2009b; Kleinstäuber et al., 2011) and three systematic reviews (Allen et al., 2002; Kleinstäuber et al., 2011; van Rood and de Roos, 2009) that focused on psychotherapies.

Three review papers focused on RCTs of CBT or behavioral medicine for somatoform disorders, medically unexplained symptoms or complaints, and somatization and somatic syndromes (Kroenke and Swindle, 2000; Looper and Kirmayer, 2002; Nezu et al., 2001). The reviews were conducted before 2007 and therefore did not include several of the individual studies described above. Two other systematic reviews looked at multiple treatments for somatoform disorders and medically unexplained symptoms (Kroenke, 2007; Sumathipala, 2007). Both concluded that the evidence supported the use of CBT more than other interventions, including pharmacologic agents, consultation letters, and exercise. All five reviews fulfill most of the criteria for Assessment of Multiple Systematic Reviews (AMSTAR) (Shea et al., 2007). Results of the five reviews all support the effectiveness of CBT and other behavioral interventions for somatic syndromes.

Abbass et al. (2009b) specifically examined psychodynamic psychotherapy for a wide variety of medically explained and unexplained disorders (for example, IBS, Crohn's disease, atopic dermatitis, and heart disease). Using AMSTAR guidance, rating categories for the quality of this are mixed. The meta-analysis conducted by Abbass et al. (2009b) showed moderate improvements for psychiatric symptoms, anxiety, and somatic symptoms. In 91.3% of the studies reviewed, short-term psychodynamic psychotherapy resulted in at least some benefit (improvement in more than one characteristic) in patients who had somatoform disorders.

A meta-analysis by Kleinstäuber et al. (2011) assessed the value of psychotherapy and showed small but consistent between-group differences in effect size and small to large within-group differences in effect size for physical symptoms and cognitive, emotional, and behavioral symptoms of somatoform disorder through the posttreatment period and follow-up. Moderator analysis for effects on physical symptoms showed that a higher number of therapy sessions was associated with better outcome. Similarly, use of therapists who are mental health professionals was associated with better outcome.

Three systematic reviews of psychotherapy interventions included such conditions as CFS, fibromyalgia, IBS, chronic pain, phantom-limb pain, psychogenic nonepileptic seizures, body dysmorphic disorder, olfactory reference syndrome, myoclonic movement, and stress-related dermatologic disorders (Allen et al., 2002; Kleinstäuber et al., 2011; van Rood and de Roos, 2009). Such aggregation of conditions makes extrapolation to CMI difficult. A review conducted by Allen et al. (2002) included only one study published since 2000 (Sumathipala et al., 2000) that was included in the present review. The van Rood and de Roos (2009) review focused on eye-movement desensitization and reprocessing (EMDR) and consisted largely of case studies. Only one study included by Russell (2008) examined EMDR for combat-related medically unexplained physical symptom; it used a single-subject case design and showed the benefit of 5 sessions of EMDR maintained through 6-month follow-up. The Russell (2008) study is not included in the present review because it does not include case studies. Accordingly, neither the van Rood and de Roos nor the Russell reviews altered the committee's conclusions.

Summary of Psychotherapy Interventions

The size of the observed effect of CBT was consistent among studies and generally in the small to moderate range. Indicators of response to interventions varied in definition among studies, and rates of response ranged from 18.5% to 60%; this suggests that although substantial gains occur in most patients, full response or remission is rare. That is similar to what happens in people who have other chronic physical and mental disorders. Review of the studies described above yields a perception that the dose of CBT may be relevant: Studies that used fewer sessions (6 or fewer) or in which CBT was delivered by a PC or a family physician rather than a mental health professional yielded less positive results (Arnold et al., 2009; Martin et al., 2007; Sumathipala et al., 2008). Similarly, the effect of the intervention may be attenuated if CBT is delivered in a group rather than individual format (Donta et al., 2003). Those factors have not been systematically evaluated. In general, attendance at treatment sessions was far from perfect but not atypical in such patient populations. Moreover, active components of the CBT interventions used in the trials have not been systematically evaluated, nor have active treatment comparisons that control for amount of patient contact been used.

The systematic reviews varied in quality and in terms of applicability to the CMI samples. There is a consensus among the committee members that somatic-focused CBT confers a consistent small to moderate effect in treatment for CMI and related somatization conditions.

On the basis of guidance provided by AHRQ (Owens et al., 2010), the committee rated the strength of evidence as shown in Table 4-5 and concluded that

- There is *high* strength of evidence of the efficacy of somatic-focused CBT for somatic-symptom syndromes. Somatic-focused individual

TABLE 4-5 Strength of Evidence on Psychotherapies

No. Studies (No. Subjects)	RoB	Consistency	Directness	Precision	Strength of Evidence
CBT, individual					
RCT: 5 (601)[a]	Low	Inconsistent	Indirect	Precise	High
Pre–post: 1 (65)[b]	High				
CBT, group					
RCT: 5 (1,531)[c]	Low	Consistent	Indirect	Precise	High
Psychodynamic, individual					
RCT: 2 (222)[d]	Moderate	Inconsistent	Indirect	Imprecise	Insufficient
Pre–post: 3 (153)[e]	High				
Psychodynamic, group					
Pre–post: 1 (40)[f]	High	N/A	Indirect	Imprecise	Insufficient

NOTES: CBT = cognitive behavioral therapy; RCT = randomized controlled trial; RoB = risk of bias.
[a]Allen et al., 2006; Escobar et al., 2007; Sharpe et al., 2011; Sumathipala et al., 2000, 2008.
[b]Arnold et al., 2009.
[c]Bleichhardt et al., 2004/Rief et al., 2002; Donta et al., 2003, and Mori et al., 2006; Lidbeck 2003; Martin et al., 2007; Zaby, 2008.
[d]Posse 2004; Sattel et al., 2012.
[e]Abbass et al., 2009a; Aiarzaguena et al., 2002; Reuber et al., 2007.
[f]Rembold, 2011.

or group CBT may be a useful intervention for veterans who have CMI.

- There is *insufficient* evidence that brief psychodynamic psycho-therapies are beneficial in treating people who have somatic syndromes. The committee draws this conclusion largely because there is not a substantial body of high-quality randomized studies, in particular studies of psychodynamic interventions alone, that is, without CBT components.

Each of the studies of psychotherapy interventions is briefly summarized in Table 4-6. Clinical trials of CBT interventions are presented first, then psychodynamic interventions, and finally systematic reviews.

MIND–BODY APPROACHES

Biofeedback

Psychophysiologic treatments comprise a set of self-regulation techniques targeted at particular symptoms or body systems. Biofeedback, the

TABLE 4-6 Psychotherapies

Study	Type	Intervention	Population
Cognitive Behavioral Therapies			
Allen et al., 2006	RCT	CBT + PCI vs PCI alone; 10 sessions over 3 months.	89% female, mean age 46.6 years, 82% white, 55% employed
Somatoform disorder			
Piscataway, New Jersey			N screened = 142 N treatment = 43 N control = 41

quintessential psychophysiologic technique, involves one or more physiologic measures (such as heart rate, muscle tension, and sweating) that target the likely pathophysiology of the patient's symptoms and teaching the patient to control his or her physiology voluntarily by watching the physiologic measures change in real time on a computer screen and developing a personal strategy for controlling them. Other components of the therapy include muscle relaxation and a self-hypnotic method called autogenic training. Psychophysiologic treatments have been found to be generally successful as treatment for various stress-related illnesses (Barrios-Choplin et al., 1997; Chappell and Chasee, 2006; McCraty et al., 1998, 2003; Reineke, 2008; Strack et al., 2004; Tanis, 2008).

The committee reviewed three studies of biofeedback in patients who had complex somatic symptoms. Two of the studies were RCTs in the United States and Germany (Katsamanis et al., 2011; Nanke and Rief, 2003), and the third one was an open trial in India (Saldanha et al., 2007).

Katsamanis et al. (2011) recruited persons who were seeking medical care for unexplained physical symptoms. People who had common disorders (such as hypertension and diabetes) were included if their personal treating physicians did not think that the physical symptoms were results of

---

Outcomes and Results

After 15 months, treatment group reported greater improvement in each outcome, and improvement increased with time (significant treatment × time interaction effects) for somatization severity, physical functioning, somatic-symptom diary, and severity of somatic symptoms. No differences at baseline.

At 15 months, severity of somatization rating (CGI for somatization disorder): CBT + PCI = 3.91 (95% CI 3.55–4.28), PCI = 4.68 (95% CI 4.32–5.05), p < 0.001; treatment × time interaction p < 0.001.

Physical functioning (SF-36): CBT + PCI = 68.57 (95% CI 60.00–77.14), PCI = 59.17 (95% CI 50.55–67.78), p = 0.01; treatment × time interaction p = 0.02.

Symptom diary: CBT + PCI = 2.59 (95% CI 2.23–2.95), PCI = 3.24 (95% CI 2.89–3.60), p = 0.002; treatment × time interaction p < 0.001.

Severity of symptoms (Severity of Somatic Symptoms Scale): CBT + PCI = 35.02 (95% CI 27.28–42.76), PCI = 45.39 (95% CI 37.66–53.12), p = 0.005; treatment × time interaction p = 0.01.

Total health care cost significantly decreased after treatment compared with control group. Median total health care costs before treatment: CBT + PCI = $1,944, PCI = $1,888; after treatment: CBT + PCI = $1,205, PCI = $1,645; p = 0.01.

No significant differences between groups in number of physician visits or diagnostic procedures.

continued

TABLE 4-6 Continued

Study	Type	Intervention	Population
Arnold et al., 2009 Somatoform disorder The Netherlands	Pre–post, controlled	CBT vs control; 5 45-min sessions over 3 months (first 4 sessions scheduled every 2 weeks, fifth planned 3 months later).	88% female, mean age 47 years, 7% unemployed or sick leave N screened = 6,409 N treatment = 31 N control = 34
Bleichhardt et al., 2004 Rief et al., 2002 Somatoform symptoms Germany	RCT Nested pre–post	CBT group therapy vs PMR group therapy vs waiting-list controls. 8 sessions of group therapy lasting 1.5 hours, 2–3 times per week over 3–4 weeks. Average treatment duration was 52 days. Individual therapy and additional group therapy for disorders (social anxiety, depression, etc.) were also provided.	73% female, mean age 44 years N PMR = 84 N soma = 107

Outcomes and Results
Only 45% (14) of participants in treatment group completed intervention; 29% (9) completed 2–4 sessions of CBT, and 26% (8) withdrew before start of treatment. According to patients' judgment of improvement, 35% of control group and 42% of treatment group had improved at 12-month follow-up (not significant). Groups did not differ significantly at baseline regarding severity of main physical symptom (measured by self-reported VAS). Recovery at 12-month follow-up (30% decrease in severity score on VAS or VAS < 5 was similar between control and treatment groups: 29% and 32%, respectively. VAS baseline to 12-month follow-up: control 7.6 (95% CI 7.2–7.9) to 6.0 (95% CI 5.2–6.8); treatment 7.6 (95% CI 7.1–8.0) to 6.0 (95% CI 5.1–6.8). Self-reported symptoms (PSC-51), anxiety and depression (HADS), functional impairment (SF-36), and illness behavior (IAS) and health care use measurements were comparable except greater mean number of physical symptoms at baseline were reported in treatment group (12.6 [95% CI 10–15]) than in control group (9.4 [95% CI 8–11]), p = 0.02. At 12-month follow-up, physical symptoms were 10.9 (95% CI 8–14) and 8.5 (95% CI 6–10) for treatment and control groups, respectively (p > 0.05).
At 1-year follow-up, significant improvements (p < 0.001) were made in all outcomes (number of symptoms, DSM-IV; general psychopathology, SCLR-90; anxiety and depression HADS; subjective health status, EQ-5D; and life satisfaction, FL2M), but there was no significant group or time × group effect. The effect of time was significant, p < 0.001, for all outcomes except no. of doctor visits in the previous year, p < 0.05. No change over 4-month waiting period was seen in controls. Mean ES for PMR = 0.57 and mean ES for the soma group = 0.67. In pre–post assessment of soma group only, at posttreatment assessments, 3 of 8 items on hourly journal evaluation had significant time effect from session 1 through session 8 ("I got suggestions for managing my symptoms," "I felt the group was helpful today," and "group atmosphere" all p < 0.05). Overall average score was about 4.0, indicating that treatment was well accepted. Motivation for psychotherapy was not a good predictor of hourly evaluations, but items for "general therapeutic experience" and "experience with respect to psychotherapy" correlated with hourly evaluations (both p < 0.01). Only controlling conviction related to hourly evaluations was "internality" (p < 0.01). Results indicate that the more positive expectations, positive previous experience, and higher internal control convictions, the more positive the hourly evaluation. After 1-year follow-up, there was significant improvement in somatic symptoms.

continued

TABLE 4-6 Continued

Study	Type	Intervention	Population
Donta et al., 2003; Mori et al., 2006 Gulf War Veterans' Illnesses (GWVI) US VA and DOD medical centers	RCT	CBT vs CBT + exercise vs exercise vs usual care. CBT was 60–90 minutes in duration; groups met weekly for 12 weeks. Aerobic exercise one 1-hour session per week with exercise therapist for 12 weeks. 2–3 independent sessions per week for 12 weeks.	15% female, mean age 41 years N screened = 2,793 N CBT + exercise = 266 N CBT only = 286 N exercise only = 269 N usual care = 271
Escobar et al., 2007 MUS New Brunswick, New Jersey	RCT	CBT vs control, 10 sessions; each 45–60 minutes long except that first session was about 90 minutes long. Sessions were delivered over 10–20 weeks with average of 3 months.	88% female, mean age 40 years, and 66% Hispanic. N screened = 416 N treatment = 87 N control = 85
Lidbeck, 1997, 2003 Functional somatic symptoms Sweden	RCT	Muscle relaxation. 8 sessions lasting for 3 hours, weekly. Administered over 2 months.	85% female, mean age 43.8 years N treatment = 33 N follow-up = 31

Outcomes and Results
At 12 months, pairwise comparisons of physical functioning (SF-36): CBT vs usual care OR 1.72 (95% CI 0.91–3.23; p value raw 0.03, corrected 0.13); CBT + exercise vs usual care OR 1.84 (95% CI 0.95–3.55; p value raw 0.02, corrected 0.09); marginal comparisons: CBT vs no CBT OR 1.71 (95% CI 1.21–2.41; p value raw 0.002, corrected 0.005). Improvement in those who attended at least 8 treatment sessions vs nonadherent patients, CBT + exercise: OR 1.71 (95% CI 0.92–3.20); CBT: OR 1.47 (95% CI 0.80–2.69; p value 0.27); exercise: OR 2.67 (95% CI 1.20–2.92). Adjusted mean change from baseline and significance compared with usual care—mental health functioning (SF-36): CBT 0.97 (p < 0.025), CBT + exercise 2.30 (p < 0.01), exercise 2.33 (p < 0.01); pain (McGill Short Form): affective pain, CBT –0.43 (p < 0.01), CBT + exercise 0.50 (p < 0.01); fatigue (MFI): general fatigue, CBT + exercise –0.97 (p < 0.01), exercise –0.87 (p < 0.01), physical fatigue, CBT + exercise –0.70 (p < 0.025), exercise –0.73 (p < 0.01); reduced activity: CBT + exercise –0.68 (p < 0.01), exercise –0.69 (p < 0.01); reduced motivation, CBT + exercise –0.35 (p < 0.025), exercise –0.38 (p < 0.01); mental fatigue, CBT + exercise –1.08 (p < 0.01), exercise –0.84 (p < 0.025); cognitive difficulties: cognition failures questionnaire, CBT 2.66 (p < 0.01), CBT + exercise 3.38 (p < 0.01), exercise 2.98 (p < 0.01); V/SF-36 mental health index, CBT + exercise 2.95 (p < 0.01), exercise 3.27 (p < 0.01); other changes for CBT, CBT + exercise, and exercise not significant.
After 6 months of follow-up, both intervention and control groups improved for all outcomes, but no significant differences between groups or group × time interactions were noted for physical functioning (SF-36 physical-functioning subscale), depression (HAM-D), anxiety (HAM-A), or medically unexplained symptoms (by visual analogue scale) except that somatic complaints (PHQ-15) were reduced in intervention group at 6 months compared with controls (p = 0.03, no interaction effect). Mean scores in treatment and control groups, respectively, from baseline to 6-month follow-up—physical functioning: 63.28–73.22 vs 61.41–69.41; somatic complaints: 14.17–9.11 vs 13.98–10.91, at 6 months p = 0.03; depression: 18.25–12.88 vs 17.41–14.29; anxiety: 20.46–14.85 vs 20.99–17.58; medically unexplained symptoms: 42.34–23.72 vs 39.62–25.25.
After 1.5 years of follow-up, significant improvement was noted for social problems (SPQ, p = 0.004), illness behavior (IBQ, p < 0.001), hypochondriasis (WI, p < 0.001), depression (HADS, p < 0.005), and anxiety (HADS, p = 0.006). Sleep quality (SDI) and medication use were most improved after treatment and then gradually worsened (both p < 0.05).

continued

TABLE 4-6 Continued

Study	Type	Intervention	Population
Martin et al., 2007 MUS Marburg, Germany	RCT	CBT vs control. CBT was administered in single session lasting 3–4 hours.	75% female, mean age 45.7 years in treatment group, 51.7 in control group N screened = 146 N treatment = 70 N control = 70
Sharpe et al., 2011 Functional (psychogenic or somatoform) symptoms Scotland	RCT	CBT-based GSH vs control. Up to 4 30-min sessions over 3 months.	71% female, mean age 43 years, 54% working N screened = 3,057 N treatment = 64 N control = 63
Sumathipala et al., 2000 Medically unexplained complaints Sri Lanka	RCT	CBT vs structured care, 6 30-min sessions over 3 months.	78% female, mean age 35 years N screened = 110 N treatment = 34 N control = 34
Sumathipala et al., 2008 MUS Sri Lanka	RCT	CBT vs control, 3 mandatory, 30-min sessions over 3 weeks; additional 3 optional sessions were offered.	79% female, mean age 34 years N screened = 504 N treatment = 75 N control = 75
Zaby et al., 2008 Somatoform symptoms Germany	RCT	CBT group therapy vs PMR group therapy vs waiting-list controls. Group interventions for CBT and PMR were 90-min weekly sessions over 8 weeks. Groups had average of 8 participants.	78% female, mean age 46.3 years N CBT = 42 N PMR = 35

Outcomes and Results

After 6 months of follow-up, both groups improved, but CBT-treated patients had greater reduction in doctor visits, medication use, and somatization (group × time interaction effect $p < 0.05$).
Outcomes at baseline to 6-month follow-up in treatment and control groups, respectively:
Health care use: mean number of doctor visits 13.4 to 8.5 vs 11.5 to 10.2, $p < 0.05$; mean days of medication use 501.9 to 398.1 vs 503.0 to 492.3, $p < 0.05$.
Somatization severity (mean BSI-somatization scale): 0.79 to 0.59 vs 0.60 to 0.61, $p < 0.05$.
Number of symptoms in last 7 days (mean SOMS-7): 9.5 to 7.8 vs 7.2 to 6.4, $p > 0.05$.
Health anxiety (mean WI): 6.5 to 5.4 vs 5.7 to 5.5, $p > 0.05$.
Global severity index (mean BSI-global severity index): 0.78 to 0.66 vs 0.61 to 0.59, $p > 0.05$.
Depression (mean BDI): 15.9 to 14.2 vs 13.2 to 11.9, $p > 0.05$.
Health-related internal control (mean KKG-I): 23.1 to 23.8 vs 22.7 to 21.8, $p < 0.10$.
Sick-leave days last month (mean): 3.8 to 1.6 vs 2.8 to 3.7, $p < 0.10$.

Treatment effects at 6-month follow-up:
Change in overall health (CGI): OR 1.5 (95% CI 0.7–2.8).
Change in presenting symptoms (CPS): OR 2.3 (95% CI 1.2–4.5).
Symptom burden (PHQ-15): mean difference –0.7 (95% CI –1.5 to 0.1).
Depression (HADS): mean difference –1.0 (95% CI –2.2 to –0.2).
Anxiety (HADS): mean difference –1.4 (95% CI –2.7 to –0.2), $p = 0.028$.
Physical functioning (SF-12): mean difference 11 (95% CI 3–19), $p = 0.008$.
Belief that symptoms are permanent: mean difference –0.5 (95% CI –0.9 to –0.1), $p = 0.024$.
Overall quality-of-care satisfaction: OR 4.0 (95% CI 1.9–8.5)

At 3-month follow-up: both groups showed improvement, but CBT-treated patients showed greater improvement.
Mean differences for psychiatric morbidity (GHQ-30) 4.1 (95% CI 0.5–7.6), $p = 0.04$; complaints 2.3 (95% CI 0.8–0.7), $p = 0.001$; number of visits 4.8 (95% CI 1.3–8), $p = 0.004$; symptoms (BSI) 2.3 (95% CI 0.5–5.2), $p = 0.01$.

At 12-month follow-up, no significant differences between CBT and structured-care interventions were reported.
Mean differences for psychiatric morbidity (GHQ-30) –0.1 (95% CI –3.3 to 3.1), $p = 0.9$; complaints 0.8 (95% CI –0.94 to 1.13), $p = 0.8$; symptoms (BSI) 0.2 (95% CI –3.1 to 3.5), $p = 0.9$; hospital visits 0.2 (95% CI –0.8 to 1.1), $p = 0.7$.

After treatment, there was significant time × group interaction over all outcomes (number and severity of somatic symptoms, SOMS-7; depression and anxiety, HADS; and health-based quality of life, SF-12 for physical and mental health). Compared with waiting controls, CBT group had fewer ($p < 0.05$) and less severe ($p < 0.01$) symptoms, improved anxiety ($p < 0.05$), and better subjective mental health ($p < 0.05$) whereas PMR group only had fewer and less severe symptoms (both $p < 0.1$). Compared with PMR, CBT showed improvement in anxiety ($p < 0.05$) and subjective mental health ($p < 0.1$).

continued

TABLE 4-6 Continued

Study	Type	Intervention	Population
Psychodynamic Therapies			
Abbass et al., 2009a MUS Halifax, Nova Scotia	Pre–post	Dynamic psychotherapy 1–25 sessions (average 3.8). Sessions were not time limited. Physician and patient collectively made decision to terminate treatment.	70% female, mean age 36.9 years N referred = 77 N enrolled = 50
Aiarzaguena et al., 2002 Somatization disorder Basque region, Spain	Pre–post	DEPENAS (a biopsychosocial intervention). Five 30-min visits conducted by 3rd-year family medicine doctors.	Age 18–65 years, mean 48 years N = 12: 9 female, 2 male, 1 uknown
Posse, 2004 Somatization Sweden	RCT	Jungian therapy vs "controls," 1 session weekly for 6 months.	N Jungian therapy = 5 N control = 5
Rembold, 2011 Somatoform disorders Germany	Pre–post, controlled	Psychosocial group therapy vs usual care. 8 1.5-hour weekly sessions, up to 10 participants per group.	75% were female. N group therapy = 20 N control = 20
Reuber et al., 2007 Functional neurologic symptoms Barnsley, United Kingdom	Pre–post	Psychotherapy. Initial "semistructured" assessment interview was 2 hours. Up to 19 sessions, each 50 min long.	81% female, mean age 44.2 years; 66.7% were "economically inactive" N referred = 94 N enrolled = 91

Outcomes and Results

After 1-year follow-up, ED visits decreased from 232 visits among all 50 participants (mean 4.6 visits/participant) 1 year before treatment to 72 (mean 1.4/patient) in year after intervention (69% reduction per participant, p < 0.001). Difference in ED visits correlated, nonsignificantly, with number of treatment sessions (Spearman r = 0.22, p = 0.13). By patient subgroups, revisit rates were reduced by 16% for all ED patients and 4.3% for patients with same symptoms as those included in study, and there was no change in ED visit rates for patients referred to study but ultimately not included in it.

Self-reported symptom outcomes: 26 patients that attended two or more sessions (mean of 5.1 treatment sessions) reported significant symptom improvement (BSI 1.21 before treatment to 0.86 after treatment, p < 0.01) and somatization subscale (1.61 before treatment to 1.04 after treatment, p = 0.02). 13 patients who completed satisfaction surveys rated treatment 7.4 of 10 on average (between "satisfied" and "very satisfied").

Significant SF-36 pre-post improvements:
Physical role functioning –25.00 to 45.45, p = 0.03.
General health perceptions –46.18 to 58.73, p = 0.003.
Emotional role functioning –54.64 to 75.73, p = 0.17.
Moderate SF-36 improvements for bodily pain –40.91 to 49.00, p = 0.03; vitality 44.09 to 51.36, p = 0.14.
Small SF-36 improvement for mental health 58.55 to 61.09, p = 0.28.

Treatment group improved more than controls in anxiety and fatigue measures (p < 0.001 or less).

Significant improvement was seen in all outcomes—number of symptoms, strength experienced and intensity of symptoms, impairment experienced because of symptoms and disease anxieties—after therapy. Frequency of PC physician visits and demand for medical tests were also reduced in treatment subjects after therapy.

---

63 patients completed median of 6 sessions (range, 1–24); 42.6% were considered by therapist to have completed treatment. Results of intent-to-treat analysis of 91 patients: After treatment, improvement (baseline to after therapy and at 6 months) was reported for all three measures of well-being (CORE-OM; 49.9 to 42.5 to 41.3, p = 0.002), physical and mental functioning (SF-36; 77.1 to 85.0 to 85.7, p < 0.001), and symptoms (PHQ-15; 13.8 to 13.0 to 12.7, p > 0.05) that were maintained after 6 months of follow-up.
Number needed to treat to improve scored by 1 SD in at least one outcome measure = 2.0; to improve 2 or more outcome measures = 3.9; and to see improvement in all 3 outcome measures = 7.0.

---

continued

TABLE 4-6 Continued

Study	Type	Intervention	Population
Sattel et al., 2012 Multisomatoform disorder	RCT	PIT vs EMC. PIT: first session was up to 90 min long; all others 45 min; 12 weekly sessions. EMC: 3 30-min sessions at 6-week intervals.	66% female, mean age 48 years; 42% were employed N screened = 662 N PIT = 107 N EMC = 104

Systematic Reviews

Abbass et al., 2009b Somatic symptom disorders Halifax, Nova Scotia	Systematic review	Short-term psychodynamic psychotherapies; models included Malan, group-analytic, Hobson, Davanloo, Luborsky, relaxation, affect-focused, group, individual, Sifneos, Strupp, Binder, body work. Number of sessions 5–22.	57.8% female, mean age 41.3 years N screened > 100 N reviewed = 23 N meta-analysis = 14
Allen et al., 2002 Multiple unexplained physical symptoms	Systematic review	Psychosocial treatments	N = 34 studies

Outcomes and Results

Average difference between PIT and EMC scores at baseline and 9-month follow-up.
Physical functioning (SF-36)—baseline: mean –0.6 (95% CI –2.43 to 1.21), p = 0.51;
9-month follow-up: mean 2.5 (0.16–5.09), p = 0.001.
Mental functioning (SF-36)—baseline: mean 0.6 (95% CI –2.85 to 3.94), 0.75; 9-month
follow-up: mean 1.1 (–2.25 to 4.55), p = 0.73.
Somatization (PHQ-15)—baseline: mean 0.4 (95% CI (–0.94 to 1.77), p = 0.48; 9-month
follow-up: mean –1.12 (–2.65 to 0.31), p = 0.01.
Depression (PHQ-15)—baseline: mean 0.5 (95% CI –1.03 to 2.06), p = 0.47; 9-month
follow-up: mean –0.8 (95% CI –2.46 to 0.90), p = 0.08.
Health Anxiety (WI)—baseline: mean –0.2 (95% CI –0.79 to 0.34), p = 0.42; 9-month
follow-up: mean –0.3 (95% CI –0.88 to 0.31), p = 0.62.
At 9-month follow-up, PIT vs EMC:
Mean number of primary care visits: 3.2 vs 3.9, p = 0.39.
Mean number of specialist consultations: 7.4 vs 7.5, p = 0.73.
% taking concurrent antidepressant medication: 36% vs 46%, p = 0.04.
% being treated with psychotherapy: 3% vs 12%, p = 0.05.

21/23 studies reported significant or possible symptom benefits related to main physical
condition; 11/12 observed significant or possible social-occupational function improvement;
16/21 observed significant or possible psychologic symptom benefits; 7 reported significant
or possible reductions in health care use. Studies included 13 medical conditions.
Meta-analyses (14 studies included): short-term (< 3 months) outcomes fixed-effect model
showed moderate improvements (ES = 0.58–0.78). There were significant (p < 0.05)
differences of moderate magnitude in medium-term (3–9 months) outcomes and long-term
(> 9 months) outcome for general psychiatric symptoms, depression, anxiety, and somatic
symptoms with the fixed-effect model (all p < 0.001). There were significant differences
(p < 0.05) of moderate magnitude in the long-term outcomes (> 9 months) with the
random-effect model.
Fixed-effect models for short-term and long-term somatic symptoms were significant (both
p < 0.0007).
Publication bias: for short-term effectiveness, N statistic range = 41–56, indicating little
publication bias; for medium term, N statistic = 16–19, indicating that results were
more subject to publication bias; for long term, N statistic = 42–44 for depression and
anxiety, but N for general psychiatric conditions = 14, and N for somatic symptoms = 12,
suggesting that results for psychiatric and somatic symptoms were more likely influenced by
publication bias than results for depression and anxiety.

No significant associations with treatment outcome were found for different diagnoses,
treatment types, treatment formats, or control conditions. Only 2 of 34 studies looked
at unexplained physical symptoms. Effect sizes were calculated for 11 studies and ranged
from 0.20 comparing dynamic therapy with standard medical care in IBS patients to 4.01
comparing EMG biofeedback with false EMD in fibromyalgia patients.

continued

TABLE 4-6 Continued

Study	Type	Intervention	Population
Kleinstäuber et al., 2011 MUPS	Systematic review	Psychotherapies, number of sessions 1–72 (mean 11). Mean therapy duration 92 days (range, 1–365 days).	72% female, mean age 44.4 years N screened = 171 N reviewed = 27
Kroenke, 2000 Somatization, somatoform disorders, persistent symptoms, or symptom syndromes	Systematic review	CBT. 24 studies used fixed number of sessions with median of 8 sessions (range, 2–16). 7 studies tailored number of sessions to patient.	N RCT = 29 N nonrandomized controlled trials = 2
Kroenke, 2007 Somatoform disorders	Systematic review		N RCTs = 34 N subjects = 3,922

Outcomes and Results
Weighted mean effect sizes for outcomes after 1 year of follow-up: Physical symptoms—between-group contrast (BGC): 0.40 (95% CI 0.1–0.7, p < 0.01); within-group contrast (WGC): 0.80 (95% CI 0.53–1.07, p < 0.001). Cognitive emotional behavioral symptoms—BGC: 0.33 (95% CI 0.17–0.5, p < 0.001); WGC: 0.57 (95% CI 0.27–0.86, p < 0.001). Depression—BGC: 0.16 (95% CI 0.02–0.30, p < 0.01); WGC: 0.40 (95% CI 0.18–0.63, p < 0.01). General psychopathology—BGC: 0.06 (95% CI −0.12 to 0.24, p = 0.5); WGC: 0.63 (95% CI 0.42–0.83, p < 0.001). Functional impairment—BGC: 0.20 (95% CI 0.05–0.34, p = 0.01); WGC: 0.42 (95% CI 0.32–0.52, p < 0.001). Health care use—BGC: 0.33 (95% CI 0.04–0.61, p < 0.05); WGC: 0.44 (95% CI 0.22–0.66, p < 0.001). On basis of 18 controlled studies, effect of psychotherapy on physical symptoms after treatment was significant (ES 0.33, 95% CI 0.23–0.43, p < 0.001). Moderator analyses showed largest effect on physical symptoms from reattribution training after follow-up (ES 0.76, 95% CI 0.46–1.06). Weighted metaregression showed that efficacy increased with more sessions in models for physical symptoms, cognitive emotional and behavioral symptoms, and depression (all p < 0.05). Authors concluded that it was unlikely that enough null-result studies were missed to decrease total weighted mean ES significantly from 0.22 to 0.05.
Most studies showed definite (71% of studies) or possible (11% of studies) treatment effect for CBT. Definite or possible treatment benefit for psychologic distress was established in 38% and 8% of 26 studies examining this outcome. Benefits of CBT regarding functional status were intermediate, showing definite or possible treatment effects in 47% (n = 9) and 26% (n = 5) of 17 studies examining this outcome. In 12 studies (3 on hypochondriasis, 2 on back pain, 2 on IBS, 1 each on CFS, chest pain, tinnitus, fibromyalgia, and unexplained somatic symptoms), patients who received CBT showed greater improvement than controls. In 6 studies (2 on back pain, 1 each on chest pain, tinnitus, electric sensitivity, and unexplained somatic symptoms), patients who received CBT did not improve more with regard to cognitive-behavioral measures.
Positive results for at least one outcome (symptoms, functional, or psychologic) were noted in 11 of 13 CBT studies and 4 of 5 antidepressants studies, whereas 8 of 16 studies of other interventions reported improvement (consultation letter to the primary care physician [4 studies], PC physician training [2 studies], and non-CBT psychotherapies [2 studies], hypnosis [2 studies], and one study each investigating multicomponent nurse-care management, aerobic exercise, writing disclosure, paradoxic intention, and explanatory therapy). CBT is most effective for variety of somatoform disorders and outcomes.

continued

TABLE 4-6 Continued

Study	Type	Intervention	Population
Looper, 2002 Somatization disorder, MUS	Systematic review	CBT; consultation letter; group therapy.	N somatization disorder = 4 studies N MUS = 5 studies
Nezu et al., 2001 MUS	Systematic review	CBT individual and group therapy. Number of sessions 4–24, 40–180 minutes.	N MUS = 9 studies
Sumathipala, 2007 Somatoform disorders	Systematic review	Miscellaneous.	N abstracts screened = 368 N systematic reviews = 6 N RCTs = 14
van Rood and de Roos, 2009 MUS	Systematic review	EMDR. Number of sessions 1–72 over 1 week–18 months.	64% female; of 57 patients with available information, average age 43 years N screened = 181 results screened N included = 16 studies (102 patients)

NOTE: BDI = Beck Depression Inventory; BSI = Brief Symptom Inventory; CBT = cognitive behavioral therapy; CFS = chronic fatigue syndrome; CGI = Clinical Global Impressions Scale; CI = confidence interval; CORE-OM = Clinical Outcomes in Routine Evaluation Outcome Measure; DEPENAS = Detection-Explanation-Plan-Exploration-Normalization-Action-Follow-Up; DSM-IV = *Diagnostic and Statistical Manual of Mental Disorders, Fourth Edition*; ED = emergency department; EMC = enhanced medical care; EMDR = eye movement desensitization and reprocessing; EQ-5D = EuroQol health status questionnaire; ES = effect size; FLZM = Questions on Life Satisfaction; GHQ-30 = 30-Item General Health Questionnaire; GSH = guided self-help; HADS = Hospital Anxiety and Depression Scale; HAM-A = Hamilton Anxiety Rating Scale; HAM-D = Hamilton Depression Rating Scale; IAS = Illness Attitude Scale; IBQ = Illness Behaviors Questionnaire; IBS = irritable bowel syndrome; MFI = Multi-

Outcomes and Results

Somatization disorder: 4 studies show consultation letters are effective in reducing excessive and expensive help-seeking associated with somatization disorder but do not improve psychologic distress of patients. Group therapy provided additional benefit not only in reducing health care costs but in improving psychologic well-being.

MUS: 3 RCTs demonstrate that individual CBT is effective in reducing somatic symptoms with effect sizes in moderate range.

Of 9 studies, only 4 met criteria allowing for calculation of effect sizes regarding efficacy of CBT. Effect-size scores for CBT ranged from 0.23 to 0.67 (mean = 0.48) for physical symptoms and 0.1 to 0.72 (mean = 0.39) for psychologic distress; this provides quantitative support for notion that CBT is effective.

Resulting studies assessed interventions that used antidepressants (1 review and 3 RCTs), CBT (5 reviews, 2 RCTs), psychiatric consultation (3 RCTs), other forms of psychotherapy (3 RCTs), exercise (2 RCTs), and collaborative care (1 RCT).

Authors note level I (systematic review) evidence that antidepressants and CBT benefit patients who have MUS, with limited level II (RCT) evidence for other interventions. No studies compared different interventions for MUS.

3 studies reported improvement in formal measures of chronic pain with decrease of 1.2–2 points (on a 10-point scale) (58 patients). Phantom-limb pain also improved (4 studies, 21 patients) by average of 4.7 points (on a 10-point scale). Another 9 studies reported clinically observed effects.

6 studies showed improvement in the form of decreased posttreatment Impact Event Scale scores compared with pretreatment score (scores decreased to nonclinical levels).

6 studies reported depression scores with BDI showing decreased score from pretreatment to posttreatment to nonclinical or mild levels.

dimensional Fatigue Inventory; MUPS = medically unexplained physical symptoms; MUS = medically unexplained symptoms; OR = odds ratio; PC = primary care; PCI = psychiatric consultation intervention; PHQ-15 = Patient Health Questionnaire 15-Item Somatic Symptom Severity Scale; PIT = psychodynamic interpersonal therapy; PMR = progressive muscle relaxation; PSC-51 = Physical Symptoms Checklist; RCT = randomized controlled trial; SCL-90-R = Symptom Checklist-90-Revised; SDI = Sleep Disturbance Inventory; SF-12 = Medical Outcomes Study 12-Item Short Form Health Survey; SF-36 = Medical Outcomes Study 36-Item Short Form Health Survey; SOMS-7 = Screening for Somatoform Symptoms-7; SPQ = Social Problems Questionnaire; V/SF-36 = Medical Outcomes Study 36-Item Short Form Health Survey for Veterans; VAS = Visual Analogue Scale; WI = Whitely Index.

underlying disorders. Participants met the abridged criteria for subthreshold somatization disorder (4 or more of a list of 42 possible somatic symptoms included in the Composite International Diagnostic Interview in men and 6 or more in women). Thirty-eight patients were randomized to the intervention or control (consultation letter) group and received an average of 10 sessions of manualized biofeedback tailored to a patient's specific symptom profile, progressive muscle relaxation, and self-hypnosis. Results showed statistically significant improvement in somatic and related symptoms in the intervention group compared with controls despite the relatively low number of patients. There was no follow-up after the intervention, so it is not known whether gains were maintained after the intervention had stopped.

Nanke et al. (2003) included patients who had diagnoses of multiple somatoform symptoms. Patients met criteria for an abridged construct of somatization, which required eight or more unexplained somatic symptoms in the *Diagnostic and Statistical Manual of Mental Disorders, Fourth Edition (DSM-IV)* list of somatic symptoms. The symptoms had to be chronic and disabling. Patients were part of a general treatment program in a hospital that consisted of CBT, physical therapy, and medical care. Fifty patients were randomly assigned to individual biofeedback or group-relaxation intervention. Outcomes focused primarily on cognitive elements ("catastrophizing") rather than somatic symptoms. After treatment, patients who received biofeedback had statistically significant improvement for catastrophizing of somatic complaints compared with patients who received group relaxation. Changes in somatic symptoms themselves and maintenance of gains after the end of the intervention were not reported.

Finally, Saldanha et al. (2007) conducted a trial of biofeedback and relaxation alone (N = 30) or jointly with pharmacotherapy (N = 30) compared with pharmacotherapy alone (N = 30) for 12 weeks and followed for up to a year in 90 participants. It does not appear that somatic symptoms were a primary target of the study inasmuch as patients who entered the study had either anxiety or depressive disorders. Patients who received biofeedback plus pharmacotherapy attained better reduction in anxiety than those on drug treatment alone or biofeedback alone, but no statistical analyses were reported.

Only Katsamanis et al. (2011) appeared to present generally low or unclear risk of bias. Although Nanke et al. (2003) used random assignment, it is unclear whether subjects or interviewers were properly blinded, so the study was judged to have a high risk of bias. Saldanha et al. (2007) also was determined to have a high risk of bias.

There have been only two controlled studies, both of which used small samples, multiple other intervention components included with biofeedback, and no follow-up. Only one of the two (Katsamanis et al., 2011) reported somatic outcomes. No studies of biofeedback targeted veterans who had CMI. On the basis of guidance provided by AHRQ (Owens et al., 2010), the committee rated the strength of evidence as shown in Table 4-7 and concluded that there is *insufficient* evidence to determine the effectiveness of biofeedback for somatic syndromes. That conclusion is largely because there is no substantial body of high-quality randomized studies in the subject. The studies of biofeedback interventions are briefly summarized in Table 4-8.

Cognitive Rehabilitation Therapy

Cognitive rehabilitation therapy (CRT) is a term used to describe a variety of interventions that have been developed to improve the cognitive function of people who have cognitive impairments. Interventions have been developed in a variety of domains—including attention, memory, processing speed, and executive function—and can be delivered individually or in a group format.

One study assessed the effect of CRT on symptoms of Gulf War syndrome in a small sample of veterans (N = 14) (Jakcsy, 2002). Slight improvements on neuropsychologic test scores were reported, but results were inconclusive because of methodologic limitations and the small sample.

On the basis of guidance provided by AHRQ (Owens et al., 2010), the committee rated the strength of evidence as shown in Table 4-9 and concluded that the evidence is *insufficient* to determine the effectiveness of CRT for symptoms of CMI in veterans. Details of Jakcsy (2002) are summarized in Table 4-10.

Complementary and Alternative Therapies

Complementary and alternative medicine (CAM) is a broad field of health care that encompasses the use of techniques to promote well-being in conjunction with conventional medicine (complementary) or in place of conventional medicine (alternative). CAM techniques to promote physical,

TABLE 4-7 Strength of Evidence on Biofeedback Interventions

No. Studies (No. Subjects)	RoB	Consistency	Directness	Precision	Strength of Evidence
RCT: 2 (88)[a] Clinical trial: 1 (90)[b]	High High	Inconsistent	Indirect	Imprecise	Insufficient

NOTES: RCT = randomized controlled trial; RoB = risk of bias.
[a]Katsamanis et al., 2011; Nanke et al., 2003.
[b]Saldanha et al., 2007.

TABLE 4-8 Biofeedback Interventions

Study	Type	Intervention	Population
Katsamanis et al., 2011 MUPS Piscataway, New Jersey	RCT	Psychophysiologic therapy (biofeedback) vs control. 10 sessions of psychophysiologic treatment over about 10 weeks.	N screened = 57 N control = 20 N treatment = 18
Nanke et al., 2003 Multiple somatoform syndrome Germany	RCT	Biofeedback vs relaxation therapy. 3 50-min sessions a week for 2 weeks.	N biofeedback = 25 N relaxation therapy = 25
Saldanha et al., 2007 Neuroses and psychosomatic disorders	Nonrandomized uncontrolled clinical trial	Biofeedback vs psychoactive drug therapy vs biofeedback and drug therapy. 5 30-min sessions a week for first 4 weeks followed by 3 30-min sessions a week for 8 weeks.	N drugs = 30 N biofeedback = 30 N drugs and biofeedback = 30

NOTE: BDI-II = Beck Depression Inventory Second Edition; CABAH = Cognitions About Body and Health Questionnaire; CGI = Clinical Global Impression Scale; MUPS = medically unexplained physical symptoms; SF-36 = Medical Outcomes Study 36-Item Short Form Health Survey; TMAS = Taylor Manifest Anxiety Scale.

Outcomes and Results
75% of the treatment group attended all 10 sessions. Estimated score change difference (p value) from baseline to final assessment (control group vs biofeedback group), corrected for age: Somatization disorder severity (CGI): −0.77, p = 0.04, d = 0.8. Depression score (BDI-II total): −5.7, p = 0.03, d = 0.81. Depression, neurovegetative subscale (BDI-II): −2.21, p = 0.045, d = 0.70. Functioning (SF-36) total: 21.57, p = 0.0011. Physical functioning (SF-36): 6.83, p = 0.0037. Mental functioning (SF-36): 8.27, p = 0.0027. Normal (SF-36): 8.18, p = 0.0009. Treatment group was significantly younger than the control group (p < 0.01).
Results revealed significant group × treatment interaction effect for reduction of "catastrophizing interpretation of bodily complaints" (CABAH, p < 0.05) but no significant effect of group or treatment alone (pretreatment and posttreatment scores, 23.1 and 19.7 vs 15.2 and 16.7, for biofeedback and relaxation, respectively) with significant reduction from baseline to posttreatment in biofeedback group (p < 0.05); no significant improvement in "intolerance of bodily complaints," "concept of bodily weakness," or "sensitivity to autonomic sensations." From baseline to posttreatment, causal attribution scores for psychosocial attribution improved in biofeedback patients (2.7 to 3.0, p < 0.01) but not relaxation patients (2.9 to 2.9, p = 0.66); significant group × treatment interaction was also found (p = 0.011). Causal attribution of symptoms to organic, genetic, and environmental factors did not change from baseline to posttreatment in either group. Sessions ratings for credibility and treatment success were significantly higher in biofeedback patients than relaxation patients (p < 0.001 and p < 0.05, respectively) and both groups' ratings improved throughout treatment (both p < 0.001). No differences in ratings of therapeutic rapport were noted.
Numbers of patients with severe (> 36), moderate (31–35), and mild (26–30) anxiety scores (TMAS) from baseline to 1 year: Drugs group: severe, 5 patients at baseline, none at follow-up; moderate, 15 patients at baseline and 5 at follow-up; mild, 10 at baseline and 17 at follow-up; no anxiety, none at baseline or follow-up (p < 0.05). Biofeedback group: severe, 4 patients at baseline and none at follow-up; moderate, 16 patients at baseline and 10 at follow-up; mild, 6 at baseline and 9 at follow-up; no anxiety, none at baseline and 4 patients at follow-up (p < 0.05). Drugs and biofeedback group: severe, 3 patients at baseline and none at follow-up; moderate, 18 patients at baseline and 3 at follow-up; mild, 8 at baseline and 6 at follow-up; no anxiety, 20 at baseline and 18 at follow-up (p < 0.02). Depression scores (BDI) at baseline and follow-up were not reported.

TABLE 4-9 Strength of Evidence on Cognitive Rehabilitation Therapies

No. Studies (No. Subjects)	RoB	Consistency	Directness	Precision	Strength of Evidence
Pre–post[a]: 1 (14)	High	N/A	Direct	Imprecise	Insufficient

NOTE: RoB = risk of bias.
[a]Jakcsy, 2002.

TABLE 4-10 Cognitive Rehabilitation Therapy

Study	Type	Intervention	Size
Jakcsy, 2002 Mild memory problems Black Hills Health Care System, VA campus at Fort Meade	Pre–post	Computer-assisted cognitive retraining vs control training, 6 4-hour sessions over 6 weeks.	Persian Gulf War veterans, 50% female, all white, average age 36 years in treatment group and 39 years in control group N eligible = 80 N treatment = 10 N control = 10

mental, and emotional well-being vary widely and include the use of natural products, such as probiotics and herbal or botanic medicines, and mind–body practices, such as acupuncture, deep-breathing techniques, yoga, and Tai Chi (NIH, 2012). The literature search found several published studies of complementary and alternative therapies, including acupuncture, movement therapies, Kampo, and St. John's wort supplements.

Acupuncture was investigated in one trial. Two publications reported on the same RCT that compared acupuncture with a control condition; Rugg et al. (2011) reported a longitudinal analysis of qualitative data, and Paterson et al. (2011) reported the quantitative results from the Classical Acupuncture Treatment for People with Unexplained Symptoms (CACTUS) study. Paterson et al. (2011) had a strong design for determining attribution, but it was not blinded. Results indicate that acupuncture improves well-being and health status. The qualitative information presented by Rugg et al. (2011) indicates that the acupuncturists in the study did a fair amount of counseling, and this leaves unclear what produced the effect. The risk of bias in the study was low.

Two of the studies assessed used body-movement-based approaches focused on a body–mind connection in psychotherapy. The study by Nickel

Outcomes and Results

Outcomes assessed 1 week to 2 months after treatment. Comparing treatment and control groups on 19 subtests to assess left hemisphere function and verbal memory and right hemisphere function and motor skills showed no significant differences in mean changes in test scores (Weschler Adult Intelligence Scale–Revised or Third Edition; Weschler Memory Scale–Revised or Third Edition; Rey Auditory Verbal Learning Test; Wisconsin Card Scoring Test; Controlled Oral Word Association Test; Porteus Mazes; Halstead Reitan Battery; and Sensory Perceptual Examination) between treatment and control groups except for Sentence Repetition Test scores (mean change scores, treatment = 4.4 and control = –5.0 , p < 0.01). Comparison of test scores on record for a cohort of normal veterans and a cohort of depressed veterans showed no significant differences in mean group scores.
14 veterans completed the study (7 in each group).

et al. (2006) included a reasonable sample size and RCT design. It was conducted on a population of 128 inpatient Turkish immigrants and found that bioenergetic exercises led to statistically significantly decreased somatization symptoms, social insecurity, depression, anxiety, hostility, anger, and tendency to direct anger inward. Payne and Stott (2010) examined the effects of dance-movement psychotherapy on 17 patients who had medically unexplained symptoms and found statistically significant increases in activity and well-being. The effect sizes were moderate to large (0.31–0.72), but the study design was poor and thus had a high risk of bias.

Beneficial effects of Kampo, an adaptation of traditional Chinese medicine, on quality of life in patients who had undifferentiated somatoform or conversion disorders were described in a poorly reported study (Yamada et al., 2005). After 3 months of Kampo, 120 subjects reported improvements in physical and psychologic health aspects of life. No information on the quality and standardization of the herbal formula was presented, and the study was judged to have a high risk of bias.

Two studies examined the potential effect of St. John's wort on somatoform disorders (Muller et al., 2004; Volz et al., 2002). Both were conducted in Germany as RCTs. Muller et al. (2004) conducted a study at a single site. Volz et al. (2002) recruited participants from 21 sites. Both studies conducted an intention-to-treat analysis with more than 150 participants. They both found consistent and fairly large effect sizes, reflecting significant improvements in anxiety and somatoform symptoms. Despite some weaknesses, both studies seem to have been rigorously conducted and to have had a low risk of bias.

On the basis of guidance provided by AHRQ (Owens et al., 2010), the committee rated the strength of evidence as shown in Table 4-11 and concluded that

- There is *low* strength of evidence that acupuncture improves well-being in people who have medically unexplained symptoms.
- There is *insufficient* evidence to support conclusions about the effectiveness of movement therapy in people who have medically unexplained symptoms or of Kampo in people who have undifferentiated somatoform disorder.
- There is *moderate* strength of evidence that St. John's wort improved symptoms in people who had somatoform disorders.

Details of each of the studies of complementary and alternative therapies are briefly summarized in Table 4-12.

TABLE 4-11 Strength of Evidence on Complementary and Alternative Therapies

No. Studies (No. Subjects)	RoB	Consistency	Directness	Precision	Strength of Evidence
Acupuncture					
RCT: 1 (80)[a]	Low	N/A	Direct	Imprecise	Low
Movement Therapy					
RCT: 1 (128)[b]	High	N/A	Indirect	Imprecise	Insufficient
Pre–post: 1 (18)[c]	High				
Kampo					
Pre–post: 1 (120)[d]	High	N/A	Indirect	Imprecise	Insufficient
St. John's Wort					
RCT: 2 (324)[e]	Low	Consistent	Direct	Precise	Moderate

NOTES: RCT = randomized controlled trial; RoB = risk of bias.
[a]Paterson et al., 2011; Rugg et al., 2011.
[b]Nickel et al., 2006.
[c]Payne and Stott, 2010.
[d]Yamada et al., 2005.
[e]Muller et al., 2004; Volz et al., 2002.

EXERCISE

Regular exercise promotes physical health, improves mood, and helps to protect from chronic diseases, such as heart disease. Exercise may also be helpful in managing a variety of illnesses (CDC, 2011).

Two studies conducted research on the effects of exercise on unexplained physical symptoms. One described the effects of CBT and exercise compared with each alone and usual care in veterans (Donta et al., 2003; Guarino et al., 2001; Mori et al., 2006). The authors showed that a combination 12-week program of group CBT and exercise led to a modest improvement in the primary outcome measure of physical function at 1 year. CBT accounted for nearly all the combined treatment effect. In contrast, almost no improvement in physical function was observed with exercise alone. The study was limited by serious lack of compliance. Only 87 (16%) attended all 12 exercise sessions, and 39 (7%) all 12 CBT sessions. How adherence with off-site exercise was monitored was not discussed. In the exercise group, participants who were adherent (attended at least eight sessions) were more than twice as likely to improve as nonadherent participants (OR 2.67, 95% CI 1.20–5.92). Even if patients were adherent, it is not clear whether the frequency and duration (1 hour per week for 12 weeks in the presence of a therapist and two or three times per week on their own) of exercise prescribed would have been adequate.

In the second study, a program of group aerobic exercise (1 hour twice a week for 10 weeks) augmented with presentation of explanatory models to link the content of training with potential amelioration of patients' symptoms reduced primary care consultations and prescriptions compared with stretching alone (Peters et al., 2002). Although there were significant improvements in both groups after 6 months, there was no difference between the two groups in patient-reported outcomes. Patient effort was titrated to maintain heart rate at 60–65% of the age-adjusted maximum, and stretching was titrated to maintain heart rate below 50% of the age-adjusted maximum.

On the basis of guidance provided by AHRQ (Owens et al., 2010), the committee rated the strength of evidence as shown in Table 4-13 and found *insufficient* evidence of the benefit of exercise in veterans who had CMI. Details of each of the studies of exercise interventions are briefly summarized in Table 4-14.

DISCUSSION

The committee encountered several difficulties when trying to make determinations of the effectiveness of treatments for CMI that precluded the drawing of conclusions with a high level of confidence. The available

TABLE 4-12 Complementary and Alternative Therapies

Study	Type	Intervention	Population
Muller et al., 2004 Unexplained multiple somatic symptoms, somatization and undifferentiated somatoform disorders, and somatoform autonomic dysfunction Germany	RCT	SJW (*Hypericum*) vs placebo. 300 mg of SJW extract administered twice daily for 6 weeks.	Treatment and control groups 60% and 76% female, respectively; mean age 47.6 years N screened = 184 N treatment = 87 N placebo = 88
Nickel et al., 2006 Chronic somatoform disorders Simbach am Inn, Germany	RCT	BE vs light gymnastics. Over 6 weeks, all patients received 2 individual psychotherapy sessions, 3 interactional group sessions, and 5 group sessions a week (all 60 mins). BE interventions were twice a week for 60 min. Control groups did light gymnastic exercise twice a week for 60 min.	About 15% of participants were Turkish immigrants; BE group mean age 48.3 years, spent 24.5 years in central Europe, and 76.6% were employed as laborers Control group mean age 49.4 years, spent 23 years in central Europe, and 71.9% were laborers N screened = 135 N treatment = 64 N control = 64
Paterson et al., 2011	RCT	Acupuncture vs waitlist. 12 60-min sessions of acupuncture over 6-month period (approximately weekly, then fortnightly, and monthly).	80% of participants female, mean age 51 years N screened = 200 N treatment = 39 N control = 41
Rugg et al., 2011 MUPS London, United Kingdom	Longitudinal qualitative interview study nested in RCT trial by Paterson et al.	Acupuncture. Two interviews lasting 45–60 min.	80% female, mean age 56 years N participants = 20

Outcomes and Results

At the end of treatment, statistically significant improvement was noted for somatic symptoms as percent change in scores from baseline to week 6 between treatment and placebo groups as measured by SOMS-7: –46.5 vs –21.5, $p \leq 0.0001$; HAM-A somatization subscale: –54.7 vs –34.0, $p \leq 0.0001$; SCL-90-R somatization subscale: –44.1 vs –15.9, $p \leq 0.0001$. Clinical improvement was also shown (CGI improvement, CGI efficacy, and global judgment of efficacy by patient, all $p \leq 0.0001$). 45.4% of treatment and 20.9% of placebo-group patients were classified as responders ($p = 0.0006$).

Tolerability and safety of SJW treatment was comparable with those of placebo. 24.1% of treatment-group patients reported total of 27 adverse events, whereas 18.1% of placebo-group patients reported total of 24 adverse events.

At end of treatment, symptom checklist (SCL-90-R) scores improved significantly more in BE than in control group for somatization (BE 75.4–64.1 vs control 74.4–69.3, $p < 0.001$), insecurity in social contexts (BE 63.5–58.1 vs control 62.4–58.7, $p = 0.02$), depression (BE 76.9–66.2 vs control 77.1–68.6, $p = 0.03$), anxiety (BE 65.3–58.1 vs control 66.1–61.1, $p = 0.04$), and hostility (BE 77.2–63.1 vs control 78.2–66.3, $p = 0.01$) but there was no significant difference in change for obsessiveness, phobic anxiety, paranoid thinking, or psychoticism. Differences in anger (measured with STAXI) were significantly greater in BE group than in control group for state anger (BE 31.9–27.3 vs control 32.2–30.7, $p = 0.01$) and anger-in (BE 26.2–18.3 vs control 22.1–20.5, $p < 0.001$). Score improved more in control group than in BE group for anger-out (BE 20.9–22.0 vs control 23.0–22.0, $p = 0.022$) with no significant difference for trait anger or anger control scores.

At 52 weeks, significant differences were noted between two groups. Adjusted mean differences for patient-reported symptoms (MYMOP) were 0.8 (95% CI 0.2–1.4), $p = 0.017$; well-being (W-BQ12) 3.8 (95% CI 1.5–6.1), $p = 0.022$; and generic outcomes (EQ-5D) 0.13 (95% CI 0.02–0.24), $p = 0.03$.

At 52 weeks, improvements in acupuncture group were maintained. Control group had received 6 months of acupuncture by this point and appeared to show a catchup improvement in all outcome measures.

"Almost all patients cited physical, psychological, and/or social changes that took place during or after their acupuncture. Some linked these directly to acupuncture, but others were unsure whether there was an association. Most of the cited changes were positive, although a few patients said that treatment had not tackled expected problems and/or didn't help at all" (Rugg et al., 2011, p. e310).

continued

TABLE 4-12 Continued

Study	Type	Intervention	Population
Payne and Stott, 2010; Payne, 2009 MUS United Kingdom	Pre–post	BMA with DMP. Four parts comprising 4 sessions lasting 2 hours each for 12 weeks.	83% of participants female, mean age 48 years N screened = 31 N enrolled = 18
Volz et al., 2002 Somatoform disorders Germany	RCT	SJW vs control. Participants received placebo or SJW tablets twice daily for 6 weeks. SJW was administered as 300-mg tablets.	72% of treatment group female, mean age 46.9 years; 62% of placebo group female, mean age 48.6 years N treatment = 75 N control = 74
Yamada et al., 2005 USD and CD Japan	Pre–post	Kampo (with supportive psychotherapy). Duration of treatment 3 months.	74% of participants female, mean age 47.1 years; 94 met criteria for USD, 26 criteria for CD N = 120

NOTES: BE = bioenergetic exercise; BMA = body–mind approach; CD = conversion disorder; CGI = Clinical Global Impressions Scale; CORE-OM = Counseling Outcome Routine Evaluation–Outcome Measure; DMP = dance-movement psychotherapy; EQ-5D = EuroQol health status questionnaire; ES = effect size; HAM-A = Hamilton Anxiety Rating Scale; MUPS = medically unexplained physical symptoms; MUS = medically unexplained symptoms; MYMOP = Measure Yourself Medical Outcome Profile; SCL-90-R = Symptom Checklist-90-Revised; SJW = St. John's wort (*Hypericum*); SOMS-7 = Screening for Somatoform Symptoms-7; STAXI = State-Trait Anger Expression Inventory; USD = undifferentiated somatiform disorder; W-BQ12 = 12-Item Well-Being Questionnaire; WHOQoL-BREF = World Health Organization Quality of Life Scale Brief Version.

Outcomes and Results

At 3-month follow-up, significant mean changes (CORE-OM, baseline to follow-up) were reported for well-being −0.76 (95% CI −1.15 to −0.38), p < 0.001, ES = 0.72; problems −0.70 (95% CI −1.13 to −0.26), p < 0.004, ES = 0.65; function −0.54 (95% CI −0.93 to −0.14), p < 0.011, ES = 0.58; risk −0.15 (95% CI −0.38 to 0.09), p < 0.204, ES = 0.31; all nonrisk −0.64 (95% CI −1.03 to −0.25), p < 0.003, ES = 0.66; all items −0.56 (−0.90 to −0.21), p < 0.003, ES = 0.66.

Significant improvements for specific symptoms were also shown (MYMOP, baseline to follow-up) for symptom one −1.7 (95% CI −2.6 to −0.8), p < 0.001, ES = 0.71; activity −2.1 (95% CI −3.4 to −0.9), p < 0.003, ES = 0.66; well-being −1.7 (95% CI −2.6 to −0.8), p < 0.001, ES = 0.71; symptom two −1.8 (95% CI −3.2 to −0.5), p < 0.012, ES = 0.67.

Facilitator and participant perceptions were compared and found to be largely congruent; participants learned how their emotions are linked to physical well-being and how to avoid or cope with symptoms in different ways.

At end of treatment, statistically significant differences were reported between treatment and control groups from day 0 to day 42 with regard to somatic anxiety (HAM-A somatization subscale SJW 15.39–6.64 vs placebo 15.55–11.97, p = 0.001), anxiety (HAM-A SJW 22.09–10.0 vs placebo 22.47–17.0, p = 0.0001), psychic anxiety (HAM-A psychic subscale SJW 6.71–3.36 vs placebo 6.92–5.03, p = 0.0001), depression (HAM-D SJW 10.59–5.43 vs placebo 10.80–8.08, p = 0.0001), psychic symptoms (SCL-90-R SJW 61.65–29.39 vs placebo 66.37–50.50, p = 0.0001), somatic symptoms (SCL-90-R somatization subscale SJW 15.57–6.84 vs placebo 15.95–12.50, p = 0.0001).

9 adverse events were observed in 8 participants in treatment group and 5 adverse events in 4 participants in control group.

After treatment, 13 participants were "very much improved," 37 "much improved," 39 "minimally improved," 9 "no change," 1 "minimally worse," and 1 "much worse." Quality-of-life (WHOQoL-BREF) score improved from 3.08 at baseline to 3.21 after 3 months (p = 0.0001). Subscores also showed significant improvement in "physical health" (p = 0.0004) and "psychological health" (p = 0.0006), and nonsignificant changes were found in "social relationships" and "environment."

Adverse events were reported in 6 patients.

TABLE 4-13 Strength of Evidence on Exercise Interventions

No. Studies (No. Subjects)	RoB	Consistency	Directness	Precision	Strength of Evidence
RCT: 2 (1,320)[a]	Intermediate	Inconsistent	Indirect	Imprecise	Insufficient

NOTES: RCT = randomized controlled trial; RoB = risk of bias.
[a]Donta et al., 2003/Mori et al., 2006; Peters et al., 2002.

TABLE 4-14 Exercise Interventions

Study	Type	Intervention	Population
Donta et al., 2003; Mori et al., 2006 Gulf War Veterans' Illnesses 18 VA and 2 DOD medical centers	RCT	CBT vs CBT + exercise. CBT was 60–90 min long; groups met weekly for 12 weeks. Aerobic exercise was one 1-hour session per week with an exercise therapist for 12 weeks and 2 or 3 independent sessions per week for 12 weeks.	Gulf War Veterans deployed August 1990 to August 1991; 15% female, mean (SD) age 40.7 (8.7) years; 24% with disability claim N screened = 2,793 N CBT + exercise = 266 N CBT only = 286 N exercise only = 269 N usual care = 271
Peters et al., 2002 PUPS Liverpool, United Kingdom	RCT	Aerobic exercise vs stretching, 1-hour sessions twice weekly for 10 weeks. Homework: exercise or stretch for 20 min 3 times weekly.	53% female, mean age 44 years (range 9–73), 46% employed N screened = 323 N aerobic training = 114 N stretching training = 114

NOTES: CBT = cognitive behavioral therapy; GP = General Practitioner; HADS = Hospital Anxiety and Depression Scale; MSPQ = Modified Somatic Perception Questionnaire; PUPS = persistent unexplained physical symptoms; RCT = randomized controlled trial; SD = standard deviation; V/SF-36 = Medical Outcomes Study 36-Item Short Form Health Survey for Veterans.

Outcomes and Results

At 12-month follow-up, physical functioning (V/SF-36): CBT + exercise adj OR = 1.84 (95% CI 0.95–3.55); CBT adj OR = 1.72 (95% CI 0.91–3.23); exercise adj OR = 1.07 (95% CI 0.63–1.82); CBT vs no CBT OR = 1.71 (95% CI 1.21–2.41); exercise vs no exercise adj OR = 1.07 (95% CI 0.76–1.50). Mean change from baseline: CBT 0.59, CBT + exercise 1.03, exercise 0.97.

Exercise alone or in combination with CBT significantly improved fatigue, cognitive symptoms, mental health functioning; CBT alone significantly improved cognitive symptoms and mental health functioning, p < 0.025. Neither had significant impact on pain.

In treatment phase, 44.9% in exercise group and 40.2% in CBT + exercise group complied (p = 0.28); in maintenance phase, 24.9% of exercise and 21.1% of CBT + exercise patients complied (p = 0.29).

6 months after training, aerobic exercise and stretching resulted in improvement from baseline with fewer symptoms recorded by GP; fewer GP consultations; fewer prescriptions; fewer secondary-care contacts; and fewer new referrals to secondary care (all p < 0.01). Anxiety and depression (HADS) and somatization (MSPQ) declined from start of program to 6-month follow-up (all p < 0.01). Reported life interference, energy, mental health, and social function improved from randomization to 6-month follow-up (all p < 0.001). No significant changes were noted in SF-36 scores. Most improvement occurred during training and did not continue in 6 months after.

No significant difference between effects of stretching and aerobic exercise on any variable. Regression models show that treatment attendance significantly reduced visits to GPs (p < 0.001), number of prescriptions (p < 0.01), number and type of prescription refills (p < 0.001) from start of treatment to 6-month follow-up but was not related to measures of symptoms and somatization.

evidence had methodologic limitations and biases that may have masked true treatment effects, and there was great diversity in study populations, types of interventions conducted, controls used, and types of outcomes assessed and measures used.

Study quality was generally poor, and samples were small (from 10 to 1,092 participants, median 87, mean 150), and many studies had high dropout rates. Most of the studies reviewed were subject to multiple sources of bias or did not clearly describe methods, and this resulted in a high proportion of studies at high or unclear risk of bias. Confounding diagnoses, such as depression and anxiety, may affect the magnitude of treatment effect and were not examined. For example, using an antidepressant to treat patients who have CMI with minor depression may improve symptoms because of changes in mood rather than changes in CMI symptoms. Some of the studies attempted to avoid that problem by excluding people who met diagnostic criteria for some psychiatric disorders or medical illnesses, but subsyndromal or undiagnosed conditions may have remained in study samples.

The heterogeneous nature of the literature limited the committee's ability to compare the efficacy of different interventions. With the exception of CBT, each intervention was the subject of only a few studies that evaluated its efficacy. The study populations were defined in different ways; some studies examined only a few symptoms not explained by medical illness, and others required diagnosis of a specific disorder for various durations and of various degrees of severity. Methods differed greatly as well: there were few blinded RCTs, and many clinical trials were influenced by varied sources of bias. The literature also used a variety of outcomes to define treatment success—such as number of symptoms, severity of symptoms, health care use, functional improvement, and changes in mood—and this made comparison difficult in that different studies used different outcomes. In addition, the numerous outcomes were measured in different ways with different tools, so comparability of studies was limited further.

Generalizability among the populations studied is questionable. Only three studies were conducted in military or veteran populations. Almost all the other study samples were dominated by middle-aged women. Thus, it is difficult to extrapolate the efficacy and acceptability of an intervention to the veteran population of interest, which is slightly younger on the average and mostly male.

Adverse effects of pharmaceuticals are typically reported, but other types of interventions may have harmful effects that are not identified or investigated. The method of adverse-event reporting may be important; use of a standardized list of adverse events may cause study participants who are suggestible (such as people who are seeking psychologic health care) to report more events than they would have otherwise (Kroenke and Rosmalen, 2006).

Length of follow-up was variable, although generally short, ranging from 1 week to 18 months (median 3 months) between the start of a study and the last assessment. Many studies collected data only immediately after treatment, whereas others assessed the effect of treatment many months after treatment had ceased.

The committee's recommendations—based on the weight of the evidence described above, treatments for comorbid and other related conditions (Chapter 5), and issues related to patient care and communication (Chapters 6 and 7)—are presented in Chapter 8.

REFERENCES

Abbass, A., S. Campbell, K. Magee, and R. Tarzwell. 2009a. Intensive short-term dynamic psychotherapy to reduce rates of emergency department return visits for patients with medically unexplained symptoms: Preliminary evidence from a pre-post intervention study. *Canadian Journal of Emergency Medical Care* 11(6):529-534.

Abbass, A., S. Kisely, and K. Kroenke. 2009b. Short-term psychodynamic psychotherapy for somatic disorders: Systematic review and meta-analysis of clinical trials. *Psychotherapy and Psychosomatics* 78(5):265-274.

AHRQ (Agency for Healthcare Research and Quality). 2011. *Effective Health Care Program. Glossary of Terms.* http://effectivehealthcare.ahrq.gov/index.cfm/glossary-of-terms/ (accessed July 1, 2012).

Aiarzaguena, J. M., G. Grandes, I. Alonso-Arbiol, J. L. del Campo Chavala, M. B. Oleaga Fernandez, and J. Marco De Juana. 2002. Bio-psychosocial treatment approach to somatizing patients in primary care: A pilot study. *Atencion Primaria* 29(9):558-561.

Allen, L. A., J. I. Escobar, P. M. Lehrer, M. A. Gara, and R. L. Woolfolk. 2002. Psychosocial treatments for multiple unexplained physical symptoms: A review of the literature. *Psychosomatic Medicine* 64(6):939-950.

Allen, L. A., R. L. Woolfolk, J. I. Escobar, M. A. Gara, and R. M. Hamer. 2006. Cognitive-behavioral therapy for somatization disorder: A randomized controlled trial. *Archives of Internal Medicine* 166(14):1512-1518.

Altamura, A. C., A. Di Rosa, A. Ermentini, G. P. Guaraldi, G. Invernizzi, N. Rudas, G. Tacchini, R. Pioli, M. T. Coppola, V. Tosini, E. Proto, E. Bolognesi, and B. Marchio. 2003. Levosulpiride in somatoform disorders: A double-blind, placebo-controlled crossover study. *International Journal of Psychiatry in Clinical Practice* 7:155-159.

Arnold, I. A., M. W. de Waal, J. A. Eekhof, W. J. Assendelft, P. Spinhoven, and A. M. van Hemert. 2009. Medically unexplained physical symptoms in primary care: A controlled study on the effectiveness of cognitive-behavioral treatment by the family physician. *Psychosomatics: Journal of Consultation Liaison Psychiatry* 50(5):515-524.

Barrios-Choplin, B., R. McCraty, and B. Cryer. 1997. An inner quality approach to reducing stress and improving physical and emotional wellbeing at work. *Stress Medicine* 13(3):193-201.

Bleichhardt, G., B. Timmer, and W. Rief. 2004. Cognitive-behavioural therapy for patients with multiple somatoform symptoms: A randomised controlled trial in tertiary care. *Journal of Psychosomatic Research* 56:449-454.

CDC (Centers for Disease Control and Prevention). 2011. *Physical Activity and Health.* http:// www.cdc.gov/physicalactivity/everyone/health/index.html (accessed September 27, 2012).

Chappell, H., and S. Chasee. 2006. The effect of biofeedback-assisted stress management training on migrant college students' anxiety and personal growth initiative. *Dissertation Abstracts International: Section B: The Sciences and Engineering* 66(11-B):62-65.

Donta, S. T., D. J. Clauw, C. C. Engel, Jr., P. Guarino, P. Peduzzi, D. A. Williams, J. S. Skinner, A. Barkhuizen, T. Taylor, L. E. Kazis, S. Sogg, S. C. Hunt, C. M. Dougherty, R. D. Richardson, C. Kunkel, W. Rodriguez, E. Alicea, P. Chiliade, M. Ryan, G. C. Gray, L. Lutwick, D. Norwood, S. Smith, M. Everson, W. Blackburn, W. Martin, J. M. Griffiss, R. Cooper, E. Renner, J. Schmitt, C. McMurtry, M. Thakore, D. Mori, R. Kerns, M. Park, S. Pullman-Mooar, J. Bernstein, P. Hershberger, D. C. Salisbury, J. R. Feussner. 2003. Cognitive behavioral therapy and aerobic exercise for Gulf War veterans' illnesses: A randomized controlled trial. *Journal of the American Medical Association* 289(11):1396-1404.

Donta, S. T., C. C. Engel, Jr., J. F. Collins, J. B. Baseman, L. L. Dever, T. Taylor, K. D. Boardman, L. E. Kazis, S. E. Martin, R. A. Horney, A. L. Wiseman, D. S. Kernodle, R. P. Smith, A. L. Baltch, C. Handanos, B. Catto, L. Montalvo, M. Everson, W. Blackburn, M. Thakore, S. T. Brown, L. Lutwick, D. Norwood, J. Bernstein, C. Bacheller, B. Ribner, L. W. P. Church, K. H. Wilson, P. Guduru, R. Cooper, J. Lentino, R. J. Hamill, A. B. Gorin, V. Gordan, D. Wagner, C. Robinson, P. DeJace, R. Greenfield, L. Beck, M. Bittner, H. R. Schumacher, F. Silverblatt, J. Schmitt, E. Wong, M. A. K. Ryan, J. Figueroa, C. Nice, J. R. Feussner. 2004. Benefits and harms of doxycycline treatment for Gulf War veterans' illnesses: A randomized, double-blind, placebo-controlled trial. *Annals of Internal Medicine* 141(2):85-94.

Escobar, J. I., M. A. Gara, A. M. Diaz-Martinez, A. Interian, M. Warman, L. A. Allen, R. L. Woolfolk, E. Jahn, and D. Rodgers. 2007. Effectiveness of a time-limited cognitive behavior therapy type intervention among primary care patients with medically unexplained symptoms. *Annals of Family Medicine* 5(4):328-335.

Fontani, V., S. Rinaldi, L. Aravagli, P. Mannu, A. Castagna, and M. L. Margotti. 2011. Noninvasive radioelectric asymmetric brain stimulation in the treatment of stress-related pain and physical problems: Psychometric evaluation in a randomized, single-blind placebo-controlled, naturalistic study. *International Journal of General Medicine* 4:681-686.

Garcia-Campayo, J., and C. Sanz-Carrillo. 2002. Topiramate as a treatment for pain in multisomatoform disorder patients: An open trial. *General Hospital Psychiatry* 24(6):417-421.

Guarino, P., P. Peduzzi, S. T. Donta, C. C. Engel, D. J. Clauw, D. A. Williams, J. S. Skinner, A. Barkhuizen, L. E. Kazis, and J. R. Feussner. 2001. A multicenter two by two factorial trial of cognitive behavioral therapy and aerobic exercise for Gulf War veterans' illnesses: Design of a Veterans Affairs cooperative study (CSP #470). *Controlled Clinical Trials* 22(3):310-332.

Han, C., C. U. Pae, B. H. Lee, Y. H. Ko, P. S. Masand, A. A. Patkar, S. H. Joe, and I. K. Jung. 2008a. Venlafaxine versus mirtazapine in the treatment of undifferentiated somatoform disorder—a 12-week prospective, open-label, randomized, parallel-group trial. *Clinical Drug Investigation* 28(4):251-261.

Han, C., D. M. Marks, C. U. Pae, B. H. Lee, Y. H. Ko, P. S. Masand, A. A. Patkar, and I. K. Jung. 2008b. Paroxetine for patients with undifferentiated somatoform disorder: A prospective, open-label, 8-week pilot study. *Current Therapeutic Research—Clinical and Experimental* 69(3):221-231.

Jakcsy, S. D. 2002. *Remediation of Acquired Memory Problems (Post War) in Gulf War Veterans Using Computer Technology.* University of Idaho.

Katsamanis, M., P. M. Lehrer, J. I. Escobar, M. A. Gara, A. Kotay, and R. Liu. 2011. Psycho-physiologic treatment for patients with medically unexplained symptoms: A randomized controlled trial. *Psychosomatics* 52(3):218-229.

Kleinstäuber, M., M. Witthoft, and W. Hiller. 2011. Efficacy of short-term psychotherapy for multiple medically unexplained physical symptoms: A meta-analysis. *Clinical Psychology Review* 31(1):146-160.

Kroenke, K. 2007. Efficacy of treatment for somatoform disorders: A review of randomized controlled trials. *Psychosomatic Medicine* 69(9):881-888.

Kroenke, K., and J. G. M. Rosmalen. 2006. Symptoms, syndromes, and the value of psychiatric diagnostics in patients who have functional somatic disorders. *Medical Clinics of North America* 90(4):603-626.

Kroenke, K., and R. Swindle. 2000. Cognitive-behavioral therapy for somatization and symptom syndromes: A critical review of controlled clinical trials. *Psychotherapy and Psychosomatics* 69(4):205-215.

Kroenke, K., N. Messina, I. Benattia, J. Graepel, and J. Musgnung. 2006. Venlafaxine extended release in the short-term treatment of depressed and anxious primary care patients with multisomatoform disorder. *Journal of Clinical Psychiatry* 67(1):72-80.

Lidbeck, J. 1997. Group therapy for somatization disorders in general practice: Effectiveness of a short cognitive-behavioural treatment model. *Acta Psychiatrica Scandinavica* 96(1):14-24.

Lidbeck, J. 2003. Group therapy for somatization disorders in primary care: Maintenance of treatment goals of short cognitive-behavioural treatment one-and-a-half-year follow-up. *Acta Psychiatrica Scandinavica* 107(6):449-456.

Looper, K. J., and L. J. Kirmayer. 2002. Behavioral medicine approaches to somatoform disorders. *Journal of Consulting & Clinical Psychology* 70(3):810-827.

Martin, A., E. Rauh, M. Fichter, and W. Rief. 2007. A one-session treatment for patients suffering from medically unexplained symptoms in primary care: A randomized clinical trial. *Psychosomatics* 48(4):294-303.

McCraty, R., B. Barrios-Choplin, D. Rozman, P. Atkinson, and A. D. Watkins. 1998. The impact of a new emotional self-management program on stress, emotions, heart rate variability, DHEA and cortisol. *Integrative Physiological and Behavioral Science* 33(2):151-170.

McCraty, R., M. Atkinson, and D. Tomasino. 2003. Impact of a workplace stress reduction program on blood pressure and emotional health in hypertensive employees. *Journal of Alternative and Complementary Medicine* 9(3):355-369.

Menza, M., M. Lauritano, L. Allen, M. Warman, F. Ostella, R. M. Hamer, and J. Escobar. 2001. Treatment of somatization disorder with nefazodone: A prospective, open-label study. *Annals of Clinical Psychiatry* 13(3):153-158.

Mori, D. L., S. Sogg, P. Guarino, J. Skinner, D. Williams, A. Barkhuizen, C. Engel, D. Clauw, S. Donta, and P. Peduzzi. 2006. Predictors of exercise compliance in individuals with Gulf War veterans illnesses: Department of Veterans Affairs cooperative study 470. *Military Medicine* 171(9):917-923.

Muller, J. E., I. Wentzel, L. Koen, D. J. Niehaus, S. Seedat, and D. J. Stein. 2008. Escitalopram in the treatment of multisomatoform disorder: A double-blind, placebo-controlled trial. *International Clinical Psychopharmacology* 23(1):43-48.

Muller, T., M. Mannel, H. Murck, and V. W. Rahlfs. 2004. Treatment of somatoform disorders with St. John's wort: A randomized, double-blind and placebo-controlled trial. *Psychosomatic Medicine* 66(4):538-547.

Nanke, A., and W. Rief. 2003. Biofeedback-based interventions in somatoform disorders: A randomized control trial. *Acta Neuropsychiatrica* 15(4):249-256.

Nezu, A. M., C. M. Nezu, and E. R. Lombardo. 2001. Cognitive-behavior therapy for medically unexplained symptoms: A critical review of the treatment literature. *Behavior Therapy* 32 (3):537-583.

Nickel, M., B. Cangoez, E. Bachler, M. Muehlbacher, N. Lojewski, N. Mueller-Rabe, F. O. Mitterlehner, P. Leiberich, N. Rother, W. Buschmann, C. Kettler, F. Pedrosa Gil, C. Lahmann, C. Egger, R. Fartacek, W. K. Rother, T. H. Loew, and C. Nickel. 2006. Bioenergetic exercises in inpatient treatment of Turkish immigrants with chronic somatoform disorders: A randomized, controlled study. *Journal of Psychosomatic Research* 61(4):507-513.

NIH (National Institutes of Health). 2012. *What Is Complementary and Alternative Medicine?* http://nccam.nih.gov/health/whatiscam (accessed September 27, 2012).

Owens, D. K., K. N. Lohr, D. Atkins, J. R. Treadwell, J. T. Reston, E. B. Bass, S. Chang, and M. Helfand. 2010. AHRQ Series Paper 5: Grading the strength of a body of evidence when comparing medical interventions: Agency for Healthcare Research and Quality and the Effective Health-Care Program. *Journal of Clinical Epidemiology* 63(5):513-523.

Paterson, C., R. S. Taylor, P. Griffiths, N. Britten, S. Rugg, J. Bridges, B. McCallum, and G. Kite. 2011. Acupuncture for "frequent attenders" with medically unexplained symptoms: A randomised controlled trial (CACTUS study). *British Journal of General Practice* 61(587):e295-305.

Payne, H., and D. Stott. 2010. Change in the moving bodymind: Quantitative results from a pilot study on the use of the bodymind approach (BMA) to psychotherapeutic group work with patients with medically unexplained symptoms (MUS). *Counselling & Psychotherapy Research* 10(4):295-306.

Peters, S., I. Stanley, M. Rose, S. Kaney, and P. Salmon. 2002. A randomized controlled trial of group aerobic exercise in primary care patients with persistent, unexplained physical symptoms. *Family Practice* 19(6):665-674.

Posse, M. 2004. Jungian psychotherapy for somatization. *European Journal of Psychiatry* 18:23-29.

Reineke, A. 2008. The effects of heart rate variability biofeedback in reducing blood pressure for the treatment of essential hypertension. *Dissertation Abstracts International: Section B: The Sciences and Engineering* 68(7-B):4880.

Rembold, S. M. E. 2011. Somatoform disorders in primary care settings: Construction and evaluation of a psychosocial group programme. *Gruppenpsychotherapie und Gruppendynamik* 47(1):2-21.

Reuber, M., C. Burness, S. Howlett, J. Brazier, and R. Grunewald. 2007. Tailored psychotherapy for patients with functional neurological symptoms: A pilot study. *Journal of Psychosomatic Research* 63(6):625-632.

Rief, W., G. Bleichhardt, and B. Timmer. 2002. Group therapy for somatoform disorders: Treatment guidelines, acceptance, and process quality. *Verhaltenstherapie* 12(3):183-191.

Rugg, S., C. Paterson, N. Britten, J. Bridges, and P. Griffiths. 2011. Traditional acupuncture for people with medically unexplained symptoms: A longitudinal qualitative study of patients' experiences. *British Journal of General Practice* 61(587):e306-e315.

Russell, M. C. 2008. War-related medically unexplained symptoms, prevalence, and treatment: Utilizing EMDR within the armed services. *Journal of EMDR Practice and Research* 2(3):212-225.

Saldanha, D., S. Chaudhury, A. A. Pawar, V. Ryali, and K. Srivastava. 2007. Reduction in drug prescription using biofeedback relaxation in neurotic and psychosomatic disorders. *Medical Journal Armed Forces India* 63(4):315-317.

Sattel, H., C. Lahmann, H. Gundel, E. Guthrie, J. Kruse, M. Noll-Hussong, C. Ohmann, J. Ronel, M. Sack, N. Sauer, G. Schneider, and P. Henningsen. 2012. Brief psychodynamic interpersonal psychotherapy for patients with multisomatoform disorder: Randomised controlled trial. *British Journal of Psychiatry* 200:60-67.

Sharpe, M., J. Walker, C. Williams, J. Stone, J. Cavanagh, G. Murray, I. Butcher, R. Duncan, S. Smith, and A. Carson. 2011. Guided self-help for functional (psychogenic) symptoms: A randomized controlled efficacy trial. *Neurology* 77(6):564-572.

Shea, B. J., J. M. Grimshaw, G. A. Wells, M. Boers, N. Andersson, C. Hamel, A. C. Porter, P. Tugwell, D. Moher, and L. M. Bouter. 2007. Development of AMSTAR: A measurement tool to assess the methodological quality of systematic reviews. *BMC Medical Research Methodology* 7(10).

Strack, B., R. Gevirtz, and W. Sime. 2004. Effect of heart rate variability (HRV) biofeedback on batting performance in baseball. *Applied Psychophysiology and Biofeedback* 29(4):299.

Sumathipala, A. 2007. What is the evidence for the efficacy of treatments for somatoform disorders? A critical review of previous intervention studies. *Psychosomatic Medicine* 69(9):889-900.

Sumathipala, A., S. Hewege, R. Hanwella, and A. H. Mann. 2000. Randomized controlled trial of cognitive behaviour therapy for repeated consultations for medically unexplained complaints: A feasibility study in Sri Lanka. *Psychological Medicine* 30(4):747-757.

Sumathipala, A., S. Siribaddana, M. Abeysingha, P. De Silva, M. Dewey, M. Prince, and A. Mann. 2008. Cognitive-behavioural therapy v. structured care for medically unexplained symptoms: Randomised controlled trial. *British Journal of Psychiatry* 193(1):51-59.

Tanis, C. 2008. The effects of heart rhythm variability biofeedback with emotional regulation on the athletic performance of women collegiate volleyball players. *Dissertation Abstracts International: Section B: Sciences and Engineering* 69(4-B):2666.

van Rood, Y. R., and C. de Roos. 2009. EMDR in the treatment of medically unexplained symptoms: A systematic review. *Journal of EMDR Practice and Research* 3(4):248-263.

Volz, H. P., H. J. Moller, I. Reimann, and K. D. Stoll. 2000. Opipramol for the treatment of somatoform disorders: Results from a placebo-controlled trial. *European Neuropsychopharmacology* 10(3):211-217.

Volz, H. P., H. Murck, S. Kasper, and H. J. Moller. 2002. St. John's wort extract (Li 160) in somatoform disorders: Results of a placebo-controlled trial. *Psychopharmacology (Berl)* 164(3):294-300.

Yamada, K., R. Den, K. Ohnishi, and S. Kanba. 2005. Effectiveness of herbal medicine (Kampo) and changes of quality of life in patients with somatoform disorders. *Journal of Clinical Psychopharmacology* 25(2):199-201.

Zaby, A., J. Heider, and A. Schroder. 2008. Waiting, relaxation, or cognitive-hehavioral therapy: How effective is outpatient group therapy for somatoform symptoms? *Zeitschrift für Klinische Psychologie und Psychotherapie* 37(1):15-23.

5

Review of Treatments for Comorbid and Related Conditions

Chronic multisymptom illness (CMI) is a serious condition that imposes an enormous burden of suffering on our nation's veterans. It can affect every facet of a veteran's health: physical, psychologic, social, economic, and spiritual; it can impair a person's capacities whether the person is a soldier, worker, or family member. Despite its impact, CMI remains poorly understood and in need of additional study. The medical community does not yet know exactly which signs and symptoms should be part of the diagnostic criteria, and, as science and discovery change, the definition and diagnostic criteria of CMI may also change.

It is known, however, that a number of events or preconditions are frequently seen in association with CMI. In some cases, a common exposure can lead to more than one condition; for example, an explosion can cause a concussion, deafness, body injury, and pain. Different but similar conditions share symptoms; for example, cognitive impairment can be a feature of CMI and traumatic brain injury (TBI). Some medical conditions can lead to other clinical problems; for example, chronic pain can lead to depression, and chronic lung disease can lead to anxiety. And some common conditions may cluster without obvious explanation. CMI may include symptoms that are not severe enough for diagnosis as a clinically recognized syndrome or that are associated with defined disorders. It is clear that the possibilities are many and that not all are fully defined.

The purpose of this report is to describe the current optimal approach to care for patients who have CMI. In the quest to help patients, the entire spectrum of their complaints must be considered and addressed. A comprehensive, individualized, patient-centered plan of care must acknowledge and address all conditions and comorbidities that are present and their possible interrelationships. This chapter briefly describes 12 common conditions that are comorbid with or related to CMI and presents treatments that are known to be effective. The committee believes that symptoms shared between CMI and those treatments may respond to similar approaches in symptom management. Treatments that are recommended in evidence-based clinical practice guidelines or that have been found effective in systematic reviews are highlighted. The chapter concludes with a general therapeutic approach to patients who have the most common diagnostic clusters.

FIBROMYALGIA

Primary fibromyalgia is a relatively common chronic condition that is thought to be caused by abnormal processing of pain by the central nervous system (Abeles et al., 2007). Using US population estimates from 2005, the estimated prevalence of fibromyalgia in the United States was about 5 million people (Lawrence et al., 2008). It is characterized by chronic widespread pain, fatigue, cognitive symptoms, and sleep disturbance. Anxiety and depression can accompany the syndrome (Wolfe et al., 1990). The diagnostic criteria of the American College of Rheumatology are as follows (Wolfe et al., 2010):

1. Pain over the preceding week identified from a list of 19 areas of the body.
2. Fatigue, waking unrefreshed, and cognitive symptoms (memory disturbance).
3. Symptoms lasting longer than 3 months.
4. Symptoms not explained by any other medical condition.

Other conditions may resemble fibromyalgia closely, including hypothyroidism, polymyalgia rheumatica, rheumatoid arthritis, and systemic lupus erythematosus.

Fibromyalgia and Chronic Multisymptom Illness

Fibromyalgia and CMI share symptoms. The hallmark of fibromyalgia is chronic widespread pain. In CMI, muscle pain and tenderness are very common but are not required for the diagnosis.

Treatments for Fibromyalgia

Many pharmacologic and nonpharmacologic treatments have been demonstrated to be effective for fibromyalgia. Many categories of pharmacologic medications are somewhat to very effective in treatment for this syndrome. Systematic reviews identified several pharmacologic treatments for fibromyalgia. Amitryptyline, a tricyclic medication, was found to have a short-term benefit—6–8 weeks—when given at 25 mg/day (Nishishinya et al., 2008). The serotonin–norepinephrine reuptake inhibitors duloxetine and milnacipran also demonstrated beneficial effects on pain reduction, fatigue, sleep, depression, and quality of life in systematic reviews (Sultan et al., 2008; Uceyler et al., 2008). The neuropathic agent pregabalin has proved to be effective (Choy et al., 2011; Nuesch et al., 2012; Siler et al., 2011; Tzellos et al., 2010). Gabapentin, another neuropathic medication, has also been shown to have modest benefits in patients who have fibromyalgia (Moore et al., 2011). Duloxetine, milnacipran, and pregabalin are approved by the US Food and Drug Administration (FDA) for the management of fibromyalgia. Other medications have shown less consistent beneficial study results, including cyclobenzaprine and the atypical analgesic tramadol (Hauser et al., 2011; Russell et al., 2000).

Nonpharmacologic interventions that have proved beneficial for patients who have fibromyalgia include cognitive behavioral therapy (CBT) (Bernardy et al., 2010) and aerobic exercise (Maquet et al., 2007). Many studies of fibromyalgia have shown benefits of multimodal therapies: a combination of treatments that include exercise, CBT, education, and self-help tools (Hauser et al., 2009). It is well established that most patients benefit from an interdisciplinary and integrative approach to the long-term management of fibromyalgia and that medications alone are rarely beneficial for maintaining effective reduction in chronic pain.

CHRONIC PAIN

Chronic pain is defined as pain that is associated with a chronic medical condition or that persists beyond the expected time for tissue healing and adversely affects the function or well-being of the person (American Society of Anesthesiologists Task Force on Chronic Pain Management and American Society of Regional Anesthesia and Pain Medicine, 2010). Chronic pain affects about 100 million adults in the United States (IOM, 2011b).

Chronic Pain and Chronic Multisymptom Illness

Chronic pain is one of the symptoms that might be associated with CMI. Veterans of the 1991 Gulf War who have CMI may not have had a specific injury but can have common and persistent diffuse chronic pain (for example, joint pain).

Pain is the most frequent presenting complaint of troops returning from the Iraq and Afghanistan wars who are treated at a VA polytrauma clinic

(Lew et al., 2009). Many Iraq and Afghanistan war veterans have chronic pain due to specific injuries. As discussed in Chapter 2, the most common health outcome reported in that population is the triad of posttraumatic stress disorder (PTSD), mild TBI, and pain (Walker et al., 2010). The prevalence of CMI in veterans of the Iraq and Afghanistan wars has not been well studied, so it is not known whether the pain reported by these veterans is associated with CMI.

Treatments for Chronic Pain

Treatment for chronic pain requires a long-term approach, coordinated care, and periodic reevaluation. The scientific literature and clinical experience support a multidisciplinary approach to treatment for chronic pain as recommended by guidelines of the American Society of Anesthesiologists Task Force on Chronic Pain Management and American Society of Regional Anesthesia and Pain Medicine (2010).

Pharmacologic management of chronic pain includes nonsteroidal anti-inflammatory drugs (NSAIDs), antidepressants, anticonvulsants, opioid therapy, and other agents. Evidence supporting pharmacologic management of chronic pain of varied etiology is strong. Tricyclic medications and serotonin–norepinephrine reuptake inhibitors (SNRIs) are recommended for chronic pain in conjunction with other therapies; there have been multiple randomized controlled trials (RCTs), and the aggregated findings are supported by meta-analyses (American Society of Anesthesiologists Task Force on Chronic Pain Management and American Society of Regional Anesthesia and Pain Medicine, 2010). Pregabalin has been shown to be effective for central neuropathic pain (Moore et al., 2009). The use of NSAIDs or tramadol for chronic back pain is supported by the results of multiple RCTs (American Society of Anesthesiologists Task Force on Chronic Pain Management and American Society of Regional Anesthesia and Pain Medicine, 2010). Although there are data that show that opioids provide effective relief of low back pain and some forms of neuropathic pain for periods ranging from 1 to 9 weeks, the data are limited with respect to the safety and efficacy of long-term opioid therapy for chronic pain. In addition, the risks and potential harm associated with opioid therapy are serious, and guidelines should be followed (VA and DOD, 2010b).

The use of radiofrequency ablation of branch nerves to facet joints for low back pain is supported by results of multiple RCTs and meta-analyses (American Society of Anesthesiologists Task Force on Chronic Pain Management and American Society of Regional Anesthesia and Pain Medicine, 2010). Ablative techniques also are recommended for neck pain, but the evidence comes from a single RCT. The use of transcutaneous electric nerve stimulation for chronic back pain and other types of pain as part of a multimodal treatment is supported by results of multiple RCTs, and the aggregated findings are supported by meta-analyses. There is no strong evidence supporting epidural injections for back pain, but there has been a single RCT on relief of leg pain. Neither is there strong evidence to support intrathecal drug therapies for neuropathic pain or minimally invasive spinal procedures for vertebral compression fractures (American Society of Anesthesiologists Task Force on Chronic Pain Management and American Society of Regional Anesthesia and Pain Medicine, 2010).

A growing body of evidence demonstrates that acupuncture can be useful for chronic pain (Lee et al., 2012; Manheimer et al., 2005; Vickers, 2012). The strongest evidence supports its use in treatment for headache, but it may be effective for other forms of chronic pain, such as low back pain and osteoarthritis. Therefore, acupuncture should be considered for use in customizing pain treatment of patients who have CMI.

CHRONIC FATIGUE SYNDROME

Chronic fatigue syndrome (CFS), also known as myalgic encephalomyelitis, affects an estimated 4 million people in the United States, according to the Centers for Disease Control and Prevention (CDC), with prevalence estimates ranging from 0.2% to 2.54% (Maquet et al., 2006; Reeves et al., 2007). CFS is more common and more severe in women and people who have Latino and African-American backgrounds, and its prognosis worsens with age (Jason et al., 2011). People who have CFS often have other comorbid conditions, such as obesity and metabolic disorders, depression, irritable bowel syndrome (IBS), fibromyalgia, and multiple chemical sensitivity. Multiple symptoms of each of those conditions can overlap substantially with CMI, including fatigue, nonrestorative sleep, tenderness on palpation, and some mild cognitive dysfunction (CDC, 1994). Definitions of CFS vary, but the diagnosis is the result of careful review of patient history, physical health and mental health examinations, clinical laboratory testing, and indicated imaging studies to rule out other medical and psychologic diagnoses that may explain the symptoms of CFS. Definitions of CFS used by CDC and UK National Health Service are included in Box 5-1.

Chronic Fatigue Syndrome and Chronic Multisymptom Illness

Much research on CFS has targeted infectious triggers associated with low-grade fever, adenopathy, and influenza symptoms. Regardless, no consistent viral agents (such as human herpesvirus 6 and Epstein-Barr virus) have been definitively identified (Glaser and Kiecolt-Glaser, 1998). Fever, adenopathy, and infection-like symptoms tend to decrease over time, and fatigue and other somatic symptoms common in CMI become more promi-

BOX 5-1
Definitions of Chronic Fatigue Syndrome

	International CFS Case Definition, 1994[a]	NICE Guidelines for CFS, 2007[b]
Duration	6 months or longer	4 months or longer in adults
Fatigue	Severe chronic fatigue not explained by any medical or psychiatric diagnosis	Fatigue with • New or specific date of onset, persistent or recurrent, unexplained by other conditions • Substantially reduced activity level • Postexertional malaise or fatigue
Symptoms	At least four of the following: • Postexertion malaise lasting more than 24 hours • Unrefreshing or nonrestorative sleep • Substantial impairment of short-term memory or concentration • Muscle pain • Pain in joints without swelling or redness • Headaches of a new type, pattern, or severity • Tender lymph nodes in the neck or armpit • Sore throat that is frequent or recurring	At least one of the following: • Difficulty in sleeping or insomnia • Muscle or joint pain without inflammation (swelling) manifested as tenderness on palpation in characteristic soft-tissue areas • Headaches • Painful lymph nodes that are not enlarged • Sore throat • Poor mental function, such as difficulty in thinking • Worsening of symptoms after physical or mental exertion • Feeling of being unwell or having influenza-like symptoms • Dizziness or nausea • Heart palpitations without heart disease
And	All other medical conditions have been ruled out.	

NOTE: CFS = chronic fatigue syndrome; NICE = National Institute for Health and Clinical Excellence.
[a]CDC, 1994.
[b]NHS, 2007.

nent (Krilov et al., 1998). Many of the symptoms of CFS and CFS-like ill-ness (meeting some but not all of the criteria for CFS) are similar to those experienced by people who have CMI. Both CMI and CFS include a variety of symptoms—fatigue, cognitive symptoms, and pain.

Treatments for Chronic Fatigue Syndrome

Both US and UK treatment guidelines emphasize the lack of a particular medication or therapy to cure CFS. However, an individualized treatment program and a patient-centered care model to tailor symptom management to a patient's needs are recommended. Symptoms of CFS may be man-aged in primary care (CDC, undated; Mayo Clinic staff, 2011; National Collaborating Centre for Primary Care, 2007).

Two specific therapies are recommended for people who have CFS: CBT and graded exercise therapy (GET) (CDC, 1994; Mayo Clinic staff, 2011; National Collaborating Centre for Primary Care, 2007). CBT provides a framework for patients to change how they think and feel about their illness and teaches behaviors that provide patients with a greater sense of control over symptoms (CDC, undated; National Collaborating Centre for Primary Care, 2007). Exercise has been associated with the body's natural release of endorphins, natural pain relievers. Both exercise and endorphins have been shown to improve a number of the symptoms of CFS and related syndromes (Cleare, 2003; Harber and Sutton, 1984).

Additional CFS management strategies can be recommended to improve quality of life. Pacing to balance activities and rest throughout the day may be helpful to avoid "crashing" after too much activity; however, evidence is insufficient to determine efficacy (CDC, 1994; National Collaborat-ing Centre for Primary Care, 2007). Disturbance of restorative or deep sleep may play a role in triggering symptoms of CFS (Moldofsky, 1993). Sleep patterns should be changed gradually to introduce a regular sleep-ing schedule, bedtime routine, noise and light control, and avoidance of caffeine, alcohol, and tobacco (CDC, 1994; National Collaborating Centre for Primary Care, 2007). Clinicians should also encourage patients to learn coping skills through counseling and support groups and to maintain their independence as much as possible (CDC, 1994; Mayo Clinic staff, 2011).

Management may focus on treating specific symptoms. Drug therapy is recommended to manage some symptoms, but clinicians are encour-aged to use as few drugs as possible and to use minimal doses because people who have CFS are often more sensitive to medications. Pain may be managed with acetaminophen, aspirin, or NSAIDs, but narcotics are not recommended. Sleep medications or treatments, such as melatonin and continuous positive airway pressure, may be useful if indicated by the patient's history and improvements are not seen with good sleep hygiene

(CDC, 1994; Mayo Clinic staff, 2011; National Collaborating Centre for Primary Care, 2007). It is clear that CFS is not depression, but it may be associated with depression.

Multivitamins can be useful for patients who do not have a balanced diet. Clinicians may offer recommendations to reduce stress and improve sleep, such as relaxation techniques and limitation of caffeine intake. Such relaxation techniques as visualization can be used to manage pain, sleep problems, and comorbid anxiety. Alternative therapies (for example, yoga, Tai Chi, acupuncture, and massage) may help to lessen pain and increase energy (CDC, 1994; Mayo Clinic staff, 2011; National Collaborating Centre for Primary Care, 2007).

SOMATIC SYMPTOM DISORDERS

There appears to be a tendency to experience and communicate psychologic distress in the form of physical symptoms and to seek medical attention for these symptoms (Katon and Walker, 1998; Shorter, 1993). Often, the physical symptoms remain medically unexplained and are associated with increased medical visits and unnecessary medical tests, which may result in iatrogenic complications. Among the many terms used in the literature to label these somatic presentations, *somatization symptoms* was the most common for decades. That designation has been gradually replaced with more descriptive terms, such as *medically unexplained symptoms, unexplained symptoms,* and *functional somatic symptoms.*

In the *Diagnostic and Statistical Manual of Mental Disorders, Fifth Edition (DSM-5)*, the new criteria being developed by the American Psychiatric Association, those syndromes are classified under the heading "Somatic Symptom Disorders" (SSDs). Their key characteristic is the presence of or preoccupation with physical symptoms that suggest a medical condition but cannot be satisfactorily explained with traditional physical and laboratory assessments (APA, 2012). *DSM-5*'s SSDs include illness anxiety disorder, functional neurologic disorder (conversion disorder), psychologic problems that affect a medical condition, and disorders not elsewhere classified. A distinctive characteristic of patients who have SSDs is not a somatic symptom itself but how a patient experiences it, interprets it, and presents it to a clinician. Despite the relevance of these somatic presentations in medicine, their definition and classification remain difficult and controversial, and this has led to frequent revisions of nomenclatures that move the target used to designate "cases" and complicate the clinical recognition and management of the syndromes.

Somatic Symptom Disorders and Chronic Multisymptom Illness

Because SSDs typically present with multiple physical symptoms of unclear etiology that tend to persist, the syndromes often overlap with CMI, and differential diagnosis is difficult.

Treatments for Somatic Symptom Disorders

Effective treatments for SSDs include nonpharmacologic approaches, such as CBT and communication with the primary care physician by the psychiatrist or psychologist via consultation letters (Escobar, 2009). Other forms of psychotherapy and biofeedback are also effective (Katsamanis et al., 2011). In some instances, particularly when SSD symptoms are accompanied by anxiety and depression symptoms (a common co-occurrence, particularly in primary care settings), such antidepressants as venlafaxine may be helpful (Kroenke et al., 2006). However, treatments have to be adapted to give proper attention to the somatic component because traditional treatments alone (for example, antidepressants) may not be sufficient.

SLEEP DISORDERS

Sleep disorders are a group of about 70 syndromes characterized by persistent disturbance in sleep that interferes with activities of daily living. The most common syndromes are chronic insomnia, nightmare disorder, rapid eye movement (REM) sleep behavior disorder, circadian-rhythm sleep disorders, and obstructive sleep apnea. Like CMI, sleep disorders are associated with fatigue, mood disturbances, cognitive difficulties, and other somatic symptoms; comorbidity with depression, anxiety, and substance abuse is common.

Sleep Disorders and Chronic Multisymptom Illness

Several types of sleep disorders are among the common symptoms associated with CMI. Nightmare disorders, subjective perceptions of difficulty with sleep initiation or duration, and early awakening (insomnia) have been described in persons who have PTSD, chronic pain disorders, and other comorbid conditions, including general medical and neurologic disorders (Chokroverty, 2000). Other types of sleep disorders are less common in people who have CMI. REM sleep behavior disorder may be idiopathic or secondary to neurologic disorders, such as Parkinson's disease, stroke, multiple sclerosis, and spinocerebellar ataxia. Obstructive sleep apnea is most common among those who are obese or have congestive heart failure, stroke, or pulmonary hypertension. Circadian-rhythm sleep dis-

TABLE 5-1 Best-Practice Guidelines and Recommendations for Treatment for Nightmare Disorders and Chronic Insomnia

Type of Intervention	Nightmare Disorder[a]	Chronic Insomnia[b]
Pharmacologic	Prazosin (for PTSD-associated nightmares)	Pharmaceutical agent selected on basis of symptom pattern, treatment goals, past treatment response, patient preference, cost, availability of other treatments, comorbid conditions, concurrent medication interactions, and side effects
Nonpharmacologic	CBT, including image rehearsal therapy	At least one behavioral intervention of these: stimulus-control therapy, relaxation therapy, or combination CBT

[a]American Academy of Sleep Medicine (Aurora et al., 2010).
[b]American Academy of Sleep Medicine (Schutte-Rodin et al., 2008).
NOTE: CBT = cognitive behavioral therapy; PTSD = posttraumatic stress disorder.

orders may be exogenous (for example, jet lag or difficulties in shift work) or endogenous (for example, advanced sleep-phase disorder or irregular sleep–wake rhythm). Nightmare disorders and insomnia are the two sleep disorders more commonly associated with CMI.

Treatments for Sleep Disorders

Because of the large number of sleep disorders and evidence that effective treatment varies among them, it is vital to evaluate the patient adequately and accurately to characterize the specific symptoms, identify potential comorbid conditions or risk factors, and diagnose the specific type of disorder. Table 5-1 summarizes best-practice guidelines and recommendations for treatment for nightmare disorder and chronic insomnia.

The clinician should consider a number of other approaches that may be useful when individualizing the treatment and management of CMI, such as good sleep hygiene, exercise, acupuncture, and mind–body approaches. Some of those approaches, such as acupuncture, have been documented with systematic reviews (Lee et al., 2012), but they have not yet risen to the level of guidelines.

FUNCTIONAL GASTROINTESTINAL DISORDERS: IRRITABLE BOWEL SYNDROME AND FUNCTIONAL DYSPEPSIA

The functional gastrointestinal disorders (FGIDs) are best understood as disorders that affect gastrointestinal functioning; the ones most recognized and most relevant to this discussion are IBS and functional dyspepsia (FD) (Drossman, 2006). IBS and FD present as recurrent or prolonged clusters of gastrointestinal symptoms that remain consistent in their features over time and among populations. IBS and FD are common in young adults and are associated with wartime deployment of Gulf War veterans (IOM, 2010).

The diagnosis of an FGID is made by fulfilling standardized symptom-based criteria ("Rome criteria") for a minimal period, usually 6 months. The criteria for IBS and FD are shown in Boxes 5-2 and 5-3.

Functional Gastrointestinal Disorders and Chronic Multisymptom Illness

The most common symptoms of IBS are abdominal pain or discomfort, diarrhea, constipation, and abdominal bloating, and common symptoms of FD are early satiety with upper abdominal fullness, burning, or pain—all in the absence of other structural abnormalities that explain the symptoms. The symptoms are common in veterans deployed to the 1991 Gulf War (IOM, 2010). There is overlap between symptoms associated with IBS and FD and the gastrointestinal symptoms associated with CMI. A veteran may fulfill criteria for IBS and also have other extraintestinal symptoms and receive a diagnosis of IBS, at another time have gastrointestinal symptoms that are not sufficient for a diagnosis of IBS, and, by virtue of having several other unexplained symptoms, be classified as having CMI. Therefore, from a therapeutic standpoint, these conditions that share symptoms are likely

---

BOX 5-2
Rome III Diagnostic Criteria[a] for Irritable Bowel Syndrome

Recurrent abdominal pain or discomfort at least 3 days per month in last 3 months associated with two or more of

1. Improvement with defecation.
2. Onset associated with a change in frequency of stool.
3. Onset associated with a change in form (appearance) of stool.

---

[a]Criteria fulfilled for the last 3 months with symptom onset at least 6 months before diagnosis.
SOURCE: Reprinted from *Gastroenterology* 130(5), Longstreth et al., Functional bowel disorders, pages 1480–1491, Copyright 2006, with permission from Elsevier.

BOX 5-3
Rome III Diagnostic Criteria[a] for Functional Dyspepsia

Must include

1. One or more of
   a. Bothersome postprandial fullness.
   b. Early satiation.
   c. Epigastric pain.
   d. Epigastric burning.
2. No evidence of structural disease (including findings of upper endoscopy) that is likely to explain the symptoms.

---

[a]Criteria fulfilled for the last 3 months with symptom onset at least 6 months before diagnosis. SOURCE: Reprinted from *Gastroenterology* 130(5), Tack et al., Functional gastroduodenal disorders, pages 1466–1479, Copyright 2006, with permission from Elsevier.

---

to respond to centrally targeted treatments that reduce symptom frequency and intensity and reduce such associated psychologic comorbidities as anxiety and depression.

Treatments for Functional Gastrointestinal Disorders

The general approach to treating IBS and FD is to look at the predominant symptom that requires treatment (for example, diarrhea, nausea, or pain) and then at the severity and intensity of the symptoms, which, when severe, are usually associated with physical and psychologic comorbidities (Drossman et al., 2002; Thiwan and Drossman, 2006).

The symptoms of IBS and FD can vary in severity. They may exist as occasional and mild gastrointestinal symptoms—which are usually treated with diet, lifestyle adjustments, or medications targeted at the bowel—or as more persistent and severe disabling symptoms that occur with other medical conditions (such as fibromyalgia, chest pain, and fatigue) and mental health conditions (such as anxiety, depression, somatization, and PTSD) that require medication targeted toward treating brain–gut dysregulation (Drossman, 2006; Drossman et al., 2002). Appendix B contains information about how brain–gut dysregulation may lead to the types of symptoms associated with IBS, FD, and CMI. The present section focuses on centrally targeted treatments because they are more applicable to treating for CMI.

Pharmacologic Treatments

The rationale for using antidepressants for IBS and FD is related to their central effects—altering pain perception; improving mood, including depression, hypervigilance, and symptom-related anxiety and increased stress reactivity; reducing associated sleep disturbances; and peripheral effects on motility and afferent signaling (Grover and Drossman, 2009). Several systematic reviews and meta-analyses have shown that antidepressants achieve both pain reduction and global symptom improvement (Chang and Drossman, 2004; Ford et al., 2009; Jackson et al., 2000; Lesbros-Pantofickova et al., 2004). The analgesic effect appears to be independent of the actions of antidepressants on mood disturbance, and a clinical response occurs before improvement in psychologic symptoms.

The authors of a systematic review concluded that tricyclic medications and the selective seratonin reuptake inhibitors (SSRIs) reduced global symptoms of IBS and abdominal pain (Ford and Vandvik, 2012). After evaluation of that and other systematic reviews and studies, tricyclic medications and SSRIs have been endorsed by the Rome Foundation (Levy et al., 2006), the American College of Gastroenterology (Brandt et al., 2009), the American Gastroenterology Association (Drossman et al., 2002), and the World Gastroenterology Organization (WGO, 2009) for treatment for IBS. More recently, some clinicians have been using SNRIs to increase adherence because they have fewer side effects than tricyclic medications.

The benefit of antidepressants for patients who have FD is less conclusive, in part because of the lack of studies of this condition, possible publication bias, and variable results primarily of small studies (Jackson et al., 2000; Mertz et al., 1998; Van Kerkhoven et al., 2008). Nevertheless, the studies are generally positive and, because of the presumed global effects of antidepressants on symptoms, these agents are commonly used in treatment for severe FD.

Nonpharmacologic Treatments

Nonpharmacologic treatments have been used commonly for many decades in treating patients who have IBS and FD because of their effects on reducing psychologic distress and their value in reducing maladaptive coping and health-related anxieties and more recently because of evidence from brain-imaging studies that they help to ameliorate symptoms (Creed et al., 2006; Rainville et al., 1999). They have synergistic effects with medical treatments, offer the advantage of few, if any, side effects, have benefits that continue after treatment, and have demonstrated a favorable cost–benefit relationship over time (Creed et al., 2006). Many treatment protocols involve a combination of relaxation and stress management with primary therapies, such as CBT or interpersonal psychotherapy. The best-designed studies have focused on CBT (Blanchard et al., 2006; Boyce et al., 2003; Drossman et al., 2003; Lackner et al., 2008) and hypnotherapy (Lindfors et al., 2012; Palsson and Whitehead, 2002; Whitehead, 2006; Whorwell et al., 1987; Wilson et al., 2006), and an abundance of robust studies have shown the benefit of both. However, whereas CBT has been very protocol-driven and can be administered by well-trained therapists in private clinical settings, hypnosis has been administered primarily in major referral centers and its efficacy in more private clinical settings is not known. A recent meta-analysis of treatments for IBS found evidence of effectiveness of CBT and hypnosis (Ford and Vandvik, 2012).

DEPRESSION

Depression is a common and disabling mood disorder. Major depressive disorder affects about 6.7% of the US population (NIH, 2012b). It is more common in women, often becomes chronic, and causes considerable impairment over the entire lifespan. Major depression is as disabling as many other chronic medical diseases, such as hypertension, congestive heart failure, and diabetes, and it adds substantial burden and disability when it appears with those disorders (Hays et al., 1995; WFMH, 2010).

The criteria for a diagnosis of major depression include the presence of mood disturbance (sadness or dysphoria) with disturbances of sleep, appetite, energy, and concentration lasting for at least 2 weeks (APA, 2000). Major depression may lead to severe complications, such as suicide. Diagnosis in primary care can be difficult because patients often present with somatic complaints and anxiety symptoms, so the diagnosis can be missed (Dowrick et al., 2005).

Depression and Chronic Multisymptom Illness

Major reasons for considering depression in veterans who have CMI are that symptoms and disabilities common in CMI (such as insomnia, fatigue, and pain in various parts of the body) are also common in severe depression and that depression is one of the clinical conditions most closely related to suicide, an outcome often reported in veterans returning from the Iraq and Afghanistan wars. Major depression often includes somatic disturbances (such as difficulty in sleeping, changes in appetite, changes in libido, and multiple aches and pains), many of which are similar to those in veterans who have CMI, so the differential diagnosis is difficult. The two syndromes can also appear together, so interventions should address both. Symptoms of major depression that are similar to those of CMI include sleep disturbance, fatigue, and pains in different parts of the body (such as headache, facial pain, and musculoskeletal pain). Like patients who have SSD, patients who have CMI often reject diagnostic assessment by mental health specialists, possibly because they perceive referral to a psychiatrist as evidence that their symptoms are not taken seriously by the treating physicians or as evidence that they are mentally ill. Proper management of CMI and depression requires a coordinated, well-integrated approach that should include medical and mental health specialists working together, ideally in a primary care setting.

Treatments for Depression

A number of treatment guidelines outline effective interventions for depression (APA, 2010; Gill et al., 2010; National Collaborating Centre for Mental Health, 2009a,b; Nieuwsma et al., 2012; Rimer et al., 2012; VA and DOD, 2009b). The most recommended treatments are non-pharmacologic approaches (such as CBT, interpersonal therapy, exercise, and acupuncture) and antidepressant medications. People who have mild to moderate depression can be treated effectively at the primary care site, often conservatively with psychotherapy and other nonpharmacologic approaches and frequent clinical monitoring and with new antidepressants (such as SSRIs) that have a good safety profile. More severe depression responds better to antidepressant medications, and at times other interventions may be needed, such as electroconvulsive therapy, particularly in severe cases that present with suicidal ideation and psychotic symptoms. Interpersonal psychotherapy alone or in combination with pharmacotherapy is effective for acute treatment for depression; interpersonal psychotherapy combined with pharmacotherapy has better response rates than pharmacotherapy alone. Several randomized clinical trials in the United States and Europe have documented the efficacy of CBT both acutely and over the long term in leading to a reduction in recurrence. CBT can be effectively implemented in nontraditional ways, such as via telephone or the Internet, to fit the needs of primary care patients.

Lithium carbonate continues to be used as an augmentation strategy, and second-generation antipsychotics—such as aripiprazole, quetiapine, and olanzapine—are used for refractory cases.

ANXIETY

Anxiety is a common symptom in patients who are seeking medical treatment. The lifetime prevalence of generalized anxiety disorder in the United States is 5.7% (NIH, 2012a). Anxiety is often a reaction to stress and is frequently associated with several chronic medical conditions, including CMI. Although anxiety may have adaptive qualities (for example, the fight-or-flight response, behavioral activation, and increased awareness), clinical or "pathologic" anxiety becomes chronic and disabling.

Pathologic anxiety is the key feature of the anxiety-disorders category, which includes many subtypes, such as panic disorder, generalized anxiety disorder, social anxiety disorder, phobic disorder, and obsessive–compulsive disorders (APA, 2000).

Diagnostic criteria for anxiety disorder include specific symptom clusters, time frames, and life courses that distinguish the various syndromes, in addition to severity, functional impairment, and symptom persistence and recurrence (APA, 2000).

Anxiety and Chronic Multisymptom Illness

Anxiety disorders are frequent in primary care, often appearing with depression and unexplained physical symptoms. They are also frequently seen in veterans (IOM, 2010) who have CMI and can be effectively recognized and treated in primary care. Generalized anxiety may be the most frequent disorder in primary care. This type of anxiety appears to be closely related to major depression, and nosologic revisions are considering combining the two diagnoses (Watson, 2005).

Treatments for Anxiety

Several guidelines and consensus documents related to treatment for anxiety disorders have been prepared by groups of experts commissioned by several professional organizations—the American Psychiatric Association (APA, 2000), the National Collaborating Centre for Primary Care (McWhinney et al., 2001), the National Institute for Health and Clinical Excellence (National Collaborating Centre for Mental Health and National Collaborating Centre for Primary Care, 2011a), and others (Sheldon et al., 2008). Briefly, the guidelines state that treatment for anxiety disorders includes a number of potential interventions, such as nonpharmacologic approaches (for example, reassurance, psychotherapy, biofeedback, relaxation, and CBT) and pharmacologic treatments (for example, antianxiety and antidepressant [SNRI] medications).

POSTTRAUMATIC STRESS DISORDER

PTSD, according to *DSM-IV-TR (Text Revision)* (APA, 2000), requires the presence of a potentially traumatic event. The person must have

- Experienced, witnessed, or been confronted by an event or events that involve actual or threatened death or serious injury or a threat to the physical integrity of oneself or others (Criterion A1), and the response must have involved intense fear, helplessness, or horror (Criterion A2).
- One or more re-experiencing symptoms (Criterion B), such as recurrent thoughts, nightmares, and flashbacks.
- Three or more avoidance or numbing symptoms (Criterion C), such as efforts to avoid thoughts, feelings, or conversations associated with the trauma; a feeling of detachment or estrangement from others; and restricted range of affect (such as being unable to have loving feelings).
- Two or more hypervigilance symptoms (Criterion D), such as difficulty in concentrating, exaggerated startle response, and irritability or outbursts of anger.

Those conditions must persist for at least 1 month (Criterion E) and cause clinically significant distress or functional impairment (Criterion F).

There are a variety of screening tools for initially assessing PTSD, including the commonly used Primary Care PTSD Screen (IOM, 2012; Prins et al., 2003). There is no evidence that one screening tool is superior to another (VA and DOD, 2010a). The Institute of Medicine (IOM, 2012) recommends that PTSD screening be conducted at least once per year when primary care clinicians see service members in Department of Defense (DOD) military treatment or at any TRICARE location, as is the case when veterans are seen in Department of Veterans Affairs (VA) facilities. If people screen positive for PTSD, the use of a structured interview, such as the Clinician-Administered PTSD Scale (Blake et al., 1995) or other structured interviews (see IOM, 2012, Table 6-3), may improve the validity and reliability of the diagnosis (IOM, 2012; VA and DOD, 2010a). Evaluation should also address comorbidities, including TBI, depression, other anxiety disorders, alcohol or substance abuse, and the presence of suicidality and risky behaviors (IOM, 2012). In summary, the diagnosis of PTSD rests on careful and comprehensive evaluation performed by a qualified professional (a psychologist, a social worker, a psychiatrist, or a psychiatric nurse-practitioner) under conditions of confidentiality (IOM, 2006).

The American Psychiatric Association is expected to release an update of *DSM*, *DSM-5*, in 2013. Proposed *DSM-5* changes include changes in Criterion A1 to add learning about an event that happened to a relative or close friend, including first responders or others who are continuously exposed to or experience details of traumatic events, and elimination of Criterion A2 because some people, such as trained military professionals, might have an emotional response during a traumatic event (Friedman et al., 2011). All 17 PTSD symptoms are proposed for retention, some with revision or regrouping. Three additional symptoms are proposed: erroneous persistent and exaggerated negative beliefs or expectations about oneself, others, or the world; persistent, distorted blame of self or others about the cause or consequences of a traumatic event; and reckless or self-destructive behavior (Friedman et al., 2011). Finally, removal of the distinction between acute and chronic is proposed. Those changes will make it necessary to update screening, self-reporting, and structured clinical instruments and to establish the reliability and validity of the altered measures.

Posttraumatic Stress Disorder and Chronic Multisymptom Illness

A number of PTSD symptoms are shared with CMI, including difficulty in falling or staying asleep, difficulty in concentrating, irritability or outbursts of anger, marked diminution of interest or participation in important activities, feeling of detachment or estrangement from others, restricted range of affect, and hypervigilance. PTSD is associated with such outcomes as lower quality of life, work-related impairment, and adverse physical health; the last is thought to be at least partially related to poor health behaviors, such as smoking, alcohol use, and physical inactivity (IOM, 2012). Somatic symptoms are commonly seen at higher rates in people who have PTSD than in trauma-exposed people who do not have PTSD and include back and neck pain, headaches, arthritis and rheumatism, chronic pain, gastrointestinal problems, and chronic fatigue (Sledjeski et al., 2008). In some cultures, PTSD often has a somatic focus including bodily heat, bodily pain, gastrointestinal distress, neck soreness, tinnitus, and orthostatic dizziness and shortness of breath (Hinton and Lewis-Fernandez, 2011).

The prevalence of PTSD was low in the 1991 Gulf War; however, veterans who had a PTSD diagnosis reported more symptoms than those who did not (Engel et al., 2000; Ford et al., 2001). Several investigations have suggested that posttraumatic stress symptoms correlate with 1991 Gulf War veterans' medically unexplained symptoms (Engel et al., 2000; Ford et al., 2001; Storzbach et al., 2000) independently of the effects of somatic or psychiatric distress, health impairment, and stress (Ford et al., 2001).

Treatments for Posttraumatic Stress Disorder

A variety of national and international PTSD treatment guidelines are based on reviews of the literature, including the VA–DOD Clinical Practice Guidelines for the Management of PTSD (VA and DOD, 2010a), the American Psychiatric Association Guideline (APA, 2004), the UK National Institute of Health and Clinical Excellence Guideline (National Collaborating Centre for Mental Health, 2005), the Australian National Health and Medical Research Council Guideline (Australian Centre for Posttraumatic Mental Health, 2007), and the International Society for Traumatic Stress Studies Guidelines (Foa et al., 2009). All the guidelines strongly support the use of trauma-focused psychologic treatment for PTSD with an emphasis on short-term trauma-focused CBT (8–12 weekly individual sessions), such as prolonged exposure or cognitive therapy (IOM, 2012). That approach is consistent with an earlier IOM (2007) conclusion that the evidence was sufficient to support the efficacy of exposure therapies in treatment for PTSD. Group-based CBT may be effective, but its outcome may not be as good as that of individual CBT (IOM, 2012).

The above guidelines are not as consistent in recommendations with regard to pharmacotherapy for PTSD, although SSRIs are generally thought to be effective (IOM, 2012). There is a lack of evidence to support complementary and alternative medicine approaches to treatment for PTSD, but a number of them are under active investigation (IOM, 2012). Accordingly, the IOM (2012) committee stated that "it is prudent to offer treatment supported by robust evidence before offering treatments that are not so supported" (p. 232). Not everyone who has PTSD responds satisfactorily to initial evidence-based treatment, although definitions of treatment response vary. The presence of psychiatric comorbidity has not been associated with worse treatment outcome and has actually been associated with better PTSD treatment outcome (Olatunji et al., 2010). For those who do not respond to first-line treatment, support for second-line and third-line interventions falls substantially and relies largely on expert clinician opinions (IOM, 2012).

TRAUMATIC BRAIN INJURY

The DOD (Helmick, 2010) defines TBI as

a traumatically induced structural injury and/or physiological disruption of brain function as a result of an external force that is indicated by new onset or worsening of a least one of the following clinical signs immediately following the event:

- Any period of loss of or decreased level of consciousness
- Any loss of memory for events immediately before or after the injury

- Any alteration in mental state at the time of injury (for example, confusion, disorientation, and slowed thinking)
- Neurological deficits (for example, weakness, loss of balance, change in vision, praxis, paresis/plegia, sensory loss, and aphasia) that may or not be transient
- Intracranial lesion. (VA and DOD, 2009a)

Severity of TBI is stratified as shown in Table 5-2.

In 2010, the Demographics and Clinical Assessment Working Group of the International and Interagency Initiative toward Common Data Elements for Research on Traumatic Brain Injury and Psychological Health simplified the definition of TBI as follows: TBI is defined as an alteration in brain function or other evidence of brain pathology caused by an external force (Menon et al., 2010). The adverse effects of concussive injury in military and civilian life have been observed increasingly, and there is increasing recognition of the importance of the proper management of this spectrum of disorders. In one sample of Army reservists returning from Iraq and Afghanistan, almost 22% screened positive for TBI (Quigley et al., 2012). The extent of exposure of deployed troops to TBI may still be underestimated.

Traumatic Brain Injury and Chronic Multisymptom Illness

People who have TBI report a large variety of physical symptoms (such as loss of balance, pain, and fatigue), cognitive symptoms (memory loss, word-finding difficulties, and reduced processing speed), and behavioral symptoms (depression, anxiety, and anger) (Gordon et al., 2000). Many of the symptoms are shared with those of CMI.

TABLE 5-2 Stratification of Severity of Traumatic Brain Injury

Mild	Moderate	Severe
Normal structural imaging	Normal or abnormal structural imaging	Normal or abnormal structural imaging
LOC for up to 30 minutes	LOC for 30 minutes to 24 hours	LOC for over 24 hours
AOC for up to 24 hours	AOC for 24 hours; severity based on other criteria	AOC for over 24 hours; severity based on other criteria
PTA for up to 1 day	PTA for 1–7 days	PTA for over 7 days

NOTES: AOC = alteration of consciousness or mental state; LOC = loss of consciousness; PTA = posttraumatic amnesia.
SOURCE: VA and DOD, 2009a.

Treatments for Traumatic Brain Injury

It is well accepted that TBI results in increased levels of depression and anxiety and in cognitive changes (Ashman et al., 2004; Hibbard et al., 1998). A systematic review completed by Fann and colleagues (2009) reported results of treatments for post-TBI depression. The largest Class I pharmacologic study found that medication did not result in a significant improvement in mood (Ashman et al., 2009). Preliminary research suggests that CBT results in an improvement in both depression and anxiety in people who have TBI (Cantor, 2011; Soo et al., 2011). There are no current guidelines for treatment for the cognitive and mood disorders experienced by people who have TBI. Cognitive rehabilitation therapy (CRT) includes a variety of treatments that have been developed to improve the cognitive function of people who have TBI. Treatments in various domains—including attention, memory, processing speed, and executive function—have been developed. They can be delivered individually or in a group format. Cicerone and colleagues in their three systematic reviews examined more than 370 studies and concluded that "there is substantial evidence to support interventions for attention, memory, social communication skills, executive function, and for comprehensive-holistic neuropsychological rehabilitation after TBI" (Cicerone et al., 2000, 2005, 2011). In contrast, an IOM committee evaluated 60 studies of the efficacy of CRT for TBI and found that although there was some benefit, the evidence was variable and insufficient overall because of many research limitations (IOM, 2011a). The committee emphasized that the lack of evidence did not mean that CRT lacks benefit, and it encouraged additional focused research. The effects of CRT on TBI depended on several factors, including the severity and the recovery phase of the injury, treatment focus and the approach used, and the outcomes measured. There was little evidence that warrants concern for potential harm or adverse events associated with CRT (IOM, 2011a).

The IOM committee concluded that CRT may help people who have cognitive deficits to compensate and improve functioning (IOM, 2011a). CRT is a flexible treatment strategy that can be administered in a variety of settings by many types of medical professionals. It may be tailored to patients' impairments, such as attention or memory problems, and approaches may be combined into a comprehensive program for patients who have multiple cognitive deficits.

SUBSTANCE-USE AND ADDICTIVE DISORDERS

DSM-IV-TR (APA, 2000) separates the constructs of substance abuse and substance dependence. The former is considered a maladaptive pattern of substance use manifested by recurrent and substantial adverse consequences related to the repeated use of the substance. The latter is considered as a cluster of cognitive, behavioral, and physiologic symptoms that indicates that a person continues to use the substance despite serious consequences, including self-administration that can result in tolerance (for example, the need for increased amounts of the substance to achieve intoxication or the desired effect or the marked diminution of the effect with continued use of the same amount of the substance), withdrawal (for example, the development of a substance-specific syndrome due to the cessation of or reduction of a substance), or compulsive drug-taking behavior. However, a large body of literature on the abuse and dependence criteria in clinical and general population samples suggests that the *DSM-IV* criteria can be considered as a unidimensional structure, with the criteria interspersed throughout the severity spectrum.

In the proposed revisions in *DSM-5*, the substance-use and addictive disorders have been reorganized according to substance; they were previously organized according to the diagnosis (that is, use, intoxication, and withdrawal) (APA, 2012). The shift will create new drug-specific categories for disorders of use of alcohol, amphetamines, cannabis, cocaine, hallucinogens, inhalants, opioids, phencyclidine, sedatives and hypnotics, stimulants and polysubstance use, and tobacco. In the reorganization, substance abuse and dependence are combined into a single disorder of graded clinical severity, for which two criteria are required for a diagnosis.

Substance-Use Disorders and Chronic Multisymptom Illness

The co-occurrence of chronic medically unexplained symptoms and substance-use disorders—including disorders of use of alcohol, opiates, and nicotine—is common (Hasin and Katz, 2007). The co-occurrence may be a relationship in itself or be due to a shared association with anxiety and depression (Regier et al., 1990). Regardless, the presence of three or more current general physical symptoms, whether medically unexplained or not, is positively associated with the likelihood of a substance-use disorder (Escobar et al., 2010). Furthermore, if chronic pain is present, there is a high likelihood of alcohol-use or nicotine-use disorder (Ekholm et al., 2009; Park et al., 2012). The medical management of chronic pain may result in the prescription of opioids because the presence of medically unexplained symptoms can interfere with the proper evaluation and management of pain. The combination of CMI and chronic pain may lead to a decision by a clinician to begin or continue opioid therapy, and use of opioids can lead to comorbidities and substance abuse or dependence, particularly in a patient who has a history of substance-use disorder. The risk of developing opioid dependence is low in patients who do not have a history of substance abuse (Friedman et al., 2003).

Treatments for Substance-Use Disorders

Pharmacotherapy

Evidence-based pharmacologic treatments are available for management of disorders of alcohol, tobacco, and opioid use. The National Institute on Drug Abuse has published *Principles of Drug Addiction Treatment: A Research-Based Guide* (NIDA, 2009), and VA and DOD have published a comprehensive clinical practice guideline that includes recommendations for evaluation of and treatment for behaviors or misuse of opiates that suggest addiction (VA and DOD, 2010b). In the case of alcohol disorders, drugs used for treatment include naltrexone (to decrease craving), acamprosate (to help in withdrawal), disulfiram (as a "negative reinforcer"), and possibly topiramate. Management options include nicotine-replacement therapy, bupropion, and varenicline for tobacco addiction and methadone, buprenorphine, and naltrexone for opioid addiction.

Psychotherapy

Evidence-based psychotherapy interventions are available for disorders of alcohol, nicotine, and opioid use. For alcohol-use disorders, behavioral couples therapy (BCT) has the strongest evidence base (Fals-Stewart et al., 2005). It is a manual-based structured therapy that combines CBT strategies with methods that address relationship issues arising from alcohol misuse and more general relationship problems with the aim of reducing distress (National Collaborating Centre for Mental Health, 2011). BCT is recommended for those who have moderate to severe alcohol dependence and should be considered for use in combination with a pharmacologic intervention.

Three other general forms of psychosocial interventions also have a strong evidence base: CBT (for example, relapse prevention, coping, and skills training), social-network and environment-based therapies (for example, cognitive behavioral strategies to build social networks that support change), and behavioral therapies (for example, cue exposure, behavioral self-control training, aversion therapy, and contingency management) (National Collaborating Centre for Mental Health, 2011). As in the case of BCT for moderate to severe dependence, combination with pharmacologic intervention should be considered. Another guideline recommends that appropriate elements of 12-step facilitation and motivational interventions should be provided as a component of assessment and intervention because the evidence is not strong enough to support their use by themselves (National Collaborating Centre for Mental Health, 2011). For nicotine addiction, both individual and group behavioral interventions focused specifically on smoking cessation, usually in combination with pharmaco-therapy, have shown evidence of being more useful than self-help strategies (Lancaster and Stead, 2008; Stead and Lancaster, 2008). For opioid users, referral to a mental health specialist is recommended by the VA–DOD guidelines if changes in mood or emotional stability are associated with nonadherent behaviors (VA and DOD, 2010b).

Other Therapies

In people with nonadherent behaviors, tapering of opioid use is safest when handled by clinicians who have expertise in pain or by a center that specializes in withdrawal treatment. It is important to include alternative strategies, such as an exercise program and psychologic support. The exercise program should be structured and include short-term goals to increase motivation to continue exercising. Family support is another key component of successful tapering off of opioid use. Educating the patient and the family about the risks associated with chronic opioid therapy, before the use of opioids, is vital.

SELF-HARM

Suicidal thoughts and ideation are typically defined as having thoughts of wanting to end one's life (AHRQ, 2004). In its diagnosis, severity of suicide risk is viewed along a continuum ranging from fleeting thoughts, such as that life is not worth living (relatively less severe), to suicidal ideation with intent and a plan (highest severity); the latter is an important risk factor in suicide attempts (AHRQ, 2004). Direct and specific questions about suicide are essential in assessment of the likelihood of suicide.

A variety of suicidality screening measures exist, including suggested questions from VA and DOD (2009c) (see Box 5-4). The ability of the screening measures to predict suicide attempts, particularly brief ones, has not been well studied (Haney et al., 2012; National Collaborating Centre for Mental Health, 2004). Patient Health Questionnaire-9 (PHQ-9) is a well-validated screening tool for assessing depression in primary care and includes one item on suicidality (Kroenke et al., 2001). In assessment, the provider should ask about suicidal thoughts, plans, and behaviors. Specific practice guidelines for assessment of risk have been developed by the American Psychiatric Association (APA, 2003), and VA has conducted a systematic review of suicide risk factors (Haney et al., 2012). Notably, primary care screening for suicide ideation among people who have signs of depression does not increase suicidal thoughts or suicide attempts (Crawford et al., 2011). A negative response to an initial question about suicidal ideation may not be enough to determine suicide risk (Jacobs and Brewer, 2006). A

BOX 5-4
Assessing for Suicidal Ideation

1. Are you discouraged about your medical condition (or social situation, etc.)?
2. Are there times when you think about your situation and feel like crying?
3. During those times, what sorts of thoughts go through your head?
4. Have you ever felt that it would not be worth living if the situation did not change (that is, have you thought about ending your life)? If so, how often do you have such thoughts?
5. Have you devised a specific plan to end your life? If so, what is your plan? If the answer is yes, do you have the necessary items to complete that plan readily available?
6. Have you ever acted on any plans to end your life in the past (that is, have you ever attempted suicide)? If the answer is yes, when did this occur? How many times has it occurred in the past? By what means? What was the outcome?

SOURCE: VA and DOD, 2009c.

---

more detailed, structured, and psychometrically validated measure to assess suicidal ideation is the Columbia-Suicide Severity Rating Scale (FDA, 2012; Posner et al., 2011), which includes items on nonsuicidal self-harm and homicidality. The objective of suicide risk assessment is to clarify the presence or absence of relevant risk and protective factors and then estimate a person's individual risk for suicide (Jacobs and Brewer, 2006).

Self-Harm and Chronic Multisymptom Illness

The presence of physical symptoms is consistently associated with suicide attempts and suicide completion. Somatization disorder is significantly associated with suicide attempts even when the effects of both a comorbid major depressive disorder and a comorbid personality disorder are controlled for; this indicates that the potential for suicide in patients who have somatization disorder should not be overlooked when a diagnosable depressive disorder or personality disorder is not present (Chioqueta and Stiles, 2004). People who completed suicide complained frequently of such somatic symptoms as gastrointestinal discomfort, headache and dizziness, and back problems during their contacts with nonpsychiatric physicians within a month before their death (Pan et al., 2009). The presence of other factors and diagnoses that often co-occur with CMI—specifically, chronic pain, activity limitations, PTSD, depression, and alcohol-use and drug-use disorders—is commonly associated with suicidality (Haney et al., 2012; Ilgen et al., 2010; US Army, 2010). Suicidality does not occur exclusively in the presence of depression (Haney et al., 2012; US Army, 2010).

Like civilian suicides, military suicides often involve problems in relationships with intimate partners, parents, or fellow unit members and tend to occur in men, who are more impulsive and use more violent means than women do (CDC, 2009; IOM, 2012). The presence of multiple stressors—including relationship, job, and physical problems—is associated with completed military suicides (Black, 2011). Three-fourths of suicide completers had contact with primary care clinicians within a year of suicide, in contrast with only one-third who had contact with mental health services. Almost half of people who committed suicide visited their physicians within a month of their death (Luoma et al., 2002). That finding is consistent with the statistic that people in military-like careers (including police and firefighting) are more prone to seek medical care because of physical than because of behavioral-health symptoms (US Army, 2010). Despite the high rate of medical contacts, most suicide completers are not identified as being at risk beforehand. Accordingly, given the association of physical symptoms with psychiatric disorders and the role of physical symptoms themselves, enhanced awareness of their link to suicide risk in nonpsychiatric settings may help to reduce suicide rates (Pan et al., 2009).

Treatments for Self-Harm

The American Psychiatric Association practice guidelines (2003) state that the documented efficacy of antidepressants in treating acute depressive episodes and their long-term benefit in patients who have recurrent forms of severe anxiety or depressive disorders support their use as part of a comprehensive care plan in people who are experiencing suicidal thoughts or behaviors. They recommend selection of an antidepressant that has a low risk of acute-overdose lethality, such as an SSRI or other newer antidepressant, and prescribing of conservative quantities, especially for patients who are not well known. Because antidepressant effects may not be observed for days or weeks after treatment starts, patients should be monitored closely early in treatment and educated about the probable delay in symptom relief (APA, 2003). There is a potential for increased risk of suicidal thoughts or behavior in children and adolescents (up to the age of 25 years) who are treated with SSRIs, although their benefit may outweigh the risk associated with them in children and adolescents who have major depression and anxiety disorders (Bridge et al., 2007). The British National

Institute of Health and Clinical Excellence clinical guidelines (National Collaborating Centre for Mental Health and National Collaborating Centre for Primary Care, 2011b) note that drug treatment should not be offered as a specific intervention to reduce self-harm and recommend considering offering 3 to 12 sessions of a psychologic intervention that is structured specifically for people who harm themselves.

Clinical consensus suggests that psychosocial interventions and specific psychotherapeutic approaches are of benefit (APA, 2003). Psychotherapies, such as interpersonal psychotherapy and CBT, that directly target self-harm (Joiner and Van Orden, 2008) may be appropriate for suicidal behavior, particularly when it occurs in the context of depression. CBT may be used to decrease two important risk factors for suicide: hopelessness and suicide attempts in depressed outpatients (APA, 2003). For patients who harm themselves repeatedly, dialectic behavior therapy, a form of CBT that teaches emotion-regulation skills, may be appropriate treatment because it is associated with decreased self-injurious behaviors, including suicide attempts (APA, 2003; National Collaborating Centre for Mental Health and National Collaborating Centre for Primary Care, 2011b).

For suicide attempters who refuse postdischarge treatment, caring letters reduce the risk of suicide (Fleischmann et al., 2008; Motto and Bostrom, 2001). Such letters are typically sent at regular intervals over at least 2 years after discharge and include a brief nondemanding statement of care, such as, "Dear ____: It has been some time since you were here at the hospital, and we hope things are going well for you. If you wish to drop us a note, we would be glad to hear from you."

GENERAL THERAPEUTIC APPROACH

In this chapter, the committee has reviewed treatments considered effective for conditions related to or comorbid with CMI. As in the case of CMI, there is ambiguity in the definitions or diagnoses of several of these conditions. However, there are shared symptoms and resulting disabilities among these conditions, as well as with CMI, and many of the treatments found to be effective for one of these conditions may be beneficial for others, including CMI. Table 5-3 shows that several treatments are considered effective in managing more than one of the related and comorbid conditions. There is substantial evidence in guidelines and from systematic reviews that tricyclic medications, SSRIs, and SNRIs may be used effectively in the management of patients who have conditions related to CMI. For example, SSRIs or SNRIs are recommended as therapy for seven of the conditions: fibromyalgia, somatic-symptom disorders, IBS, anxiety, depression (including depression resulting from chronic pain or CFS), PTSD, and self-harm.

TABLE 5-3 Summary of Treatments Recommended in Guidelines or Found to Be Effective in Systematic Reviews for Conditions Comorbid with and Related to Chronic Multisymptom Illness

Condition	Pharmacologic	Nonpharmacologic
Fibromyalgia	• SNRIs (duloxetine and milnacipram) • Tricyclic medication (amitriptyline) • Pregabalin • Gabapentin	• CBT • Aerobic exercise • Combination of exercise, CBT, education, and self-help books
Chronic pain	• Tricyclic medications • SNRIs and SSRIs • NSAIDs • Anticonvulsants • Opioids	• Radiofrequency ablation of medial branch nerves to facet joints for low back pain • Acupuncture for headaches and low back pain • Transcutaneous electric nerve stimulation for temporary relief of low back pain • Epidural steroids for leg pain • Physical or restorative therapy • Psychologic treatment (for example, CBT, biofeedback, relaxation training) • Botulinum-toxin injections for chronic migraines
Chronic fatigue syndrome	• NSAIDs for pain symptoms • Melatonin for problems in sleeping • Antidepressants for depression and to improve sleep quality	• CBT • Graded exercise therapy • Lifestyle changes (for example, regular sleeping schedule; avoidance of caffeine, alcohol, and tobacco; and dietary changes) • Alternative therapies (for example, yoga, Tai Chi, acupuncture, and massage) • CPAP for problems in sleeping
Somatic-symptom disorders	• SNRI (venlafaxine) if anxiety and depression symptoms are present	• CBT and other forms of psychotherapy • Biofeedback • Consultation letters to primary-care physicians

TABLE 5-3 Continued

Condition	Pharmacologic	Nonpharmacologic
Sleep disorders	• For nightmare disorder, prazosin • For chronic insomnia, select pharmaceutical agent on basis of symptom pattern, treatment goals, past treatment response, patient preference, cost, availability of other treatments, comorbid conditions, concurrent medication interactions, and side effects	• For nightmare disorder, CBT, including image rehearsal therapy • For chronic insomnia, stimulus-control therapy or relaxation therapy, or combination CBT
Irritable bowel syndrome	• Tricyclic medications • SSRIs and SNRIs	• CBT • Hypnosis
Functional dyspepsia	No treatments identified	
Depression	• Tricyclic medications • SSRIs	• CBT • Interpersonal therapy • Exercise • Acupuncture • Electroconvulsive therapy (for severe depression only)
Anxiety	• Antianxiety medications • SSRIs	• CBT • Reassurance • Psychotherapy • Relaxation
Posttraumatic stress disorder	• SSRIs	• CBT
Traumatic brain injury	No treatments identified	• CBT

continued

TABLE 5-3 Continued

Condition	Pharmacologic	Nonpharmacologic
Substance-use and addictive disorders	For alcohol-use disorders: • Naltrexone • Acamprosate • Disulfiram • Topiramate (possibly) For tobacco-use disorders: • Nicotine-replacement therapy • Bupropion • Varenicline For opioid-use disorders: • Methadone • Buprenorphine • Naltrexone	For alcohol-use disorders: • Behavioral couples therapy • CBT • Social network and environment-based therapies • Other behavioral therapies (for example, cue exposure, behavioral self-control training, aversion therapy, and contingency management) For tobacco-use disorders: • Individual and group behavioral interventions focused on smoking cessation For opioid-use disorders: • Referral to a pain specialist or center that specializes in withdrawal treatment
Self-harm	• SSRIs	• CBT, including dialectic behavior therapy • Interpersonal therapy

NOTES: CBT = cognitive behavioral therapy; CPAP = continuous positive airway pressure; NSAIDs = nonsteroidal anti-inflammatory drugs; SNRIs = serotonin–norepinephrine reuptake inhibitors; SSRIs = selective serotonin reuptake inhibitors.

There also is substantial evidence in guidelines and from systematic reviews that CBT is effective in managing more than one of the related conditions. CBT has been shown to be effective in nearly all the conditions examined in this chapter. It is important to note that there are multiple types of CBT and that the choice of the appropriate type to use for a particular patient will depend on the person's symptoms.

As summarized in this chapter, many other treatments, both pharmacologic and nonpharmacologic, have been shown to be effective in managing conditions related to and comorbid with CMI. Because symptoms of CMI have a pattern of presentation similar to those of the other conditions, treatments found to be effective for the conditions should be considered as parts of an integrated and multimodal treatment plan for patients who have CMI.

REFERENCES

Abeles, A. M., M. H. Pillinger, B. M. Solitar, and M. Abeles. 2007. Narrative review: The pathophysiology of fibromyalgia. *Annals of Internal Medicine* 146(10):726-734.

AHRQ (Agency for Healthcare Research and Quality). 2004. *Screening for Suicide Risk: A Systematic Evidence Review for the U.S. Preventive Task Force.* Rockville, MD. http://www.ahrq.gov/downloads/pub/prevent/pdfser/suicidser.pdf (accessed November 13, 2012).

American Society of Anesthesiologists Task Force on Chronic Pain Management and American Society of Regional Anesthesia and Pain Medicine. 2010. Practice guidelines for chronic pain management. *Anesthesiology* 112(4):810-833.

APA (American Psychiatric Association). 2000. *Diagnostic and Statistical Manual of Mental Disorders, IV.* Washington, DC: APA.

APA. 2003. *Practice Guidelines for the Assessment and Treatment of Patients with Suicidal Behaviors.* http://psychiatryonline.org/content.aspx?bookid=28&sectionid=1673332 (accessed November 13, 2012).

APA. 2004. *Practice Guidelines for Treatment of PTSD and Acute Stress Disorder.* http://psychiatryonline.org/content.aspx?bookid=28&sectionid=1670530 (accessed November 13, 2012).

APA. 2010. *Practice Guidelines for the Treatment of Patients with Major Depressive Disorder.* http://psychiatryonline.org/data/Books/prac/PG_Depression3rdEd.pdf (accessed November 13, 2012).

APA. 2012. *DSM-5 Development.* http://www.dsm5.org/Pages/Default.aspx (accessed November 13, 2012).

Ashman, T. A., L. A. Spielman, M. R. Hibbard, J. M. Silver, T. Chandna, and W. A. Gordon. 2004. Psychiatric challenges in the first 6 years after traumatic brain injury: Cross-sequential analyses of Axis I disorders. *Archives of Physical Medicine and Rehabilitation* 85(4):S36-S42.

Ashman, T. A., J. B. Cantor, W. A. Gordon, S. Flanagan, A. Ginsberg, C. Engmann, L. A. Spielman, M. Egan, A. F. Ambrose, and B. Greenwald. 2009. A randomized controlled trial of setraline for the treatment of depression in individuals with traumatic brain injury. *Archives of Physical Medicine & Rehabilitation* 90:733-740.

Aurora, R. N., R. S. Zak, S. H. Auerbach, K. R. Casey, S. Chowdhuri, A. Karippot, R. K. Maganti, K. Ramar, D. A. Kristo, S. R. Bista, C. I. Lamm, and T. I. Morgenthaler. 2010. Best practice guide for the treatment of nightmare disorder in adults. *Journal of Clinical Sleep Medicine* 6(4):389-401.

Australian Centre for Posttraumatic Mental Health. 2007. *Australian Guidelines for the Treatment of Adults with Acute Stress Disorder and Posttraumatic Stress Disorder.* Melbourne, Australia: National Health and Medical Research Council. http://www.nhmrc.gov.au/_files_nhmrc/publications/attachments/mh13.pdf (accessed November 13, 2012).

Bernardy, K., N. Fuber, V. Kollner, and W. Hauser. 2010. Efficacy of cognitive-behavioral therapies in fibromyalgia syndrome: A systematic review and metaanalysis of randomized controlled trials. *Journal of Rheumatology* 37(10):1991-2005.

Black, S. A. 2011. Prevalence and risk factors associated with suicides in Army soldiers. *Military Psychology* 23:433-451.

Blake, D. D., F. W. Weathers, L. M. Nagy, D. G. Kaloupek, F. D. Gusman, D. S. Charney, and T. M. Keane. 1995. The development of a clinician-administered PTSD scale. *Journal of Traumatic Stress* 8(1):75-90.

Blanchard, E. B., J. M. Lackner, R. Gusmano, G. D. Gudleski, K. Sanders, L. Keefer, and S. Krasner. 2006. Prediction of treatment outcome among patients with irritable bowel syndrome treated with group cognitive therapy. *Behaviour Research and Therapy* 44(3):317-337.

Boyce, P. M., N. J. Talley, B. Balaam, N. A. Koloski, and G. Truman. 2003. A randomized controlled trial of cognitive behavior therapy, relaxation training, and routine clinical care for the irritable bowel syndrome. *American Journal of Gastroenterology* 98(10):2209-2218.

Brandt, L. J., W. D. Chey, A. E. Foxx-Orenstein, E. M. M. Quigley, L. R. Schiller, P. S. Schoenfeld, B. M. Spiegel, N. J. Talley, and P. Moayyedi. 2009. An evidence-based position statement on the management of irritable bowel syndrome. *American Journal of Gastroenterology* 104:S1-S36.

Bridge, J. A., S. Iyengar, C. B. Salary, R. P. Barbe, B. Birmaher, H. A. Pincus, L. Ren, and D. A. Brent. 2007. Clinical response and risk for reported suicidal ideation and suicide attempts in pediatric antidepressant treatment: A meta-analysis of randomized controlled trials. *Journal of the American Medical Association* 297(15):1683-1696.

Cantor, J. B. 2011. *A Randomized Controlled Trial of Psychotherapies for Post-TBI Depression: Initial Findings, A Presentation.* Paper presented at American Congress of Rehabilitation Medicine.

CDC (Centers for Disease Control and Prevention). 1994. *Chronic Fatigue Syndrome: The 1994 Case Definition.* http://www.cdc.gov/cfs/case-definition/1994.html (accessed November 13, 2012).

CDC. 2009. *Suicide: Facts at a Glance.* http://www.cdc.gov/ViolencePrevention/pdf/Suicide-DataSheet-a.pdf (accessed Septmeber 27, 2012).

CDC. Undated. *Chronic Fatigue Syndrome: A Tool Kit for Providers.* http://www.cdc.gov/cfs/pdf/cfs-toolkit.pdf (accessed November 13, 2012).

Chang, L., and D. A. Drossman. 2004. Psychotropic drugs and management of patients with functional gastrointestinal disorders. *Advanced Therapy in Gastroenterology and Liver Disease.* Hamilton, Ontario: BC Decker.

Chioqueta, A. P., and T. C. Stiles. 2004. Suicide risk in patients with somatization disorder. *The Journal of Crisis Intervention and Suicide Prevention* 25:3-7.

Chokroverty, S. 2000. Diagnosis and treatment of sleep disorders caused by co-morbid disease. *Neurology* 54(5 Suppl 1):S8-S15.

Choy, E., D. Marshall, Z. L. Gabriel, S. A. Mitchell, E. Gylee, and H. A. Dakin. 2011. A systematic review and mixed treatment comparison of the efficacy of pharmacological treatments for fibromyalgia. *Seminars in Arthritis and Rheumatism* 41(3):335-345.

Cicerone, K. D., C. Dahlberg, K. Kalmar, D. M. Langenbahn, J. F. Malec, T. F. Bergquist, T. Felicetti, J. T. Giacino, J. P. Harley, D. E. Harrington, J. Herzog, S. Kneipp, L. Laatsch, and P. A. Morse. 2000. Evidence-based cognitive rehabilitation: Recommendations for clinical practice. *Archives of Physical Medicine and Rehabilitation* 81(12):1596-1615.

Cicerone, K. D., C. Dahlberg, J. F. Malec, D. M. Langenbahn, T. Felicetti, S. Kneipp, W. Ellmo, K. Kalmar, J. T. Giacino, J. P. Harley, L. Laatsch, P. A. Morse, and J. Catanese. 2005. Evidence-based cognitive rehabilitation: Updated review of the literature from 1998 through 2002. *Archives of Physical Medicine and Rehabilitation* 86(8):1681-1692.

Cicerone, K. D., D. M. Langenbahn, C. Braden, J. F. Malec, K. Kalmar, M. Fraas, T. Felicetti, L. Laatsch, J. P. Harley, T. Bergquist, J. Azulay, J. Cantor, and T. Ashman. 2011. Evidence-based cognitive rehabilitation: Updated review of the literature from 2003 through 2008. *Archives of Physical Medicine and Rehabilitation* 92(4):519-530.

Cleare, A. J. 2003. The neuroendocrinology of chronic fatigue syndrome. *Endocrine Reviews* 24(2):236-252.

Crawford, M. J., L. Thana, C. Methuen, P. Ghosh, S. V. Stanley, J. Ross, F. Gordon, G. Blair, and P. Bajaj. 2011. Impact of screening for risk of suicide: Randomised controlled trial. *British Journal of Psychiatry* 198(5):379-384.

Creed, F., R. L. Levy, L. A. Bradley, C. Fransisconi, D. A. Drossman, and B. D. Naliboff. 2006. Psychosocial aspects of functional gastrointestinal disorders. In *Rome III: The Functional Gastrointestinal Disorders.* 3rd ed, edited by D. A. Drossman, E. Corazziari, M. Delvaux, R. C. Spiller, N. J. Talley and W. G. Thompson. McLean, VA: Degnon Associates, Inc. Pp. 295-368.

Dowrick, C., C. Katona, R. Peveler, and H. Lloyd. 2005. Somatic symptoms and depression: Diagnostic confusion and clinical neglect. *British Journal of General Practice* 55(520):829-830.

Drossman, D. A. 2006. The functional gastrointestinal disorders and the Rome III process. In *Rome III: The Functional Gastrointestinal Disorders.* 3rd ed, edited by D. A. Drossman, E. Corazziari, M. Delvaux, R. Spiller, N. J. Talley and W. G. Thompson. McLean, VA: Degnon Associates, Inc. Pp. 1-29.

Drossman, D. A., M. Camilleri, E. A. Mayer, and W. E. Whitehead. 2002. AGA technical review on irritable bowel syndrome. *Gastroenterology* 123(6):2108-2131.

Drossman, D. A., B. B. Toner, W. E. Whitehead, N. E. Diamant, C. B. Dalton, S. Duncan, S. Emmott, V. Proffitt, D. Akman, K. Frusciante, T. Le, K. Meyer, B. Bradshaw, K. Mikula, C. B. Morris, C. J. Blackman, Y. M. Hu, H. G. Jia, J. Z. Li, G. G. Koch, and S. I. Bangdiwala. 2003. Cognitive-behavioral therapy versus education and desipramine versus placebo for moderate to severe functional bowel disorders. *Gastroenterology* 125(1):19-31.

Ekholm, O., M. Gronbaek, V. Peuckmann, and P. Sjogren. 2009. Alcohol and smoking behavior in chronic pain patients: The role of opioids. *European Journal of Pain* 13(6):606-612.

Engel, C. C., Jr., X. Liu, B. D. McCarthy, R. F. Miller, and R. Ursano. 2000. Relationship of physical symptoms to posttraumatic stress disorder among veterans seeking care for Gulf War-related health concerns. *Psychosomatic Medicine* 62(6):739-745.

Escobar, J. 2009. Somatoform disorders. In *Kaplan and Sadock's Comprehensive Textbook of Psychiatry.* 9th ed, edited by B. J. Sadock, V. A. Sadock and P. Ruiz. Philadelphia: Lippincott Williams & Wilkins.

Escobar, J. I., B. Cooke, C. N. Chen, M. A. Gara, M. Alegria, A. Interian, and E. Diaz. 2010. Whether medically unexplained or not, three or more concurrent somatic symptoms predict psychopathology and service use in community populations. *Journal of Psychosomatic Research* 69(1):1-8.

Fals-Stewart, W., T. J. O'Farrell, G. R. Birchler, J. Cordova, and M. L. Kelley. 2005. Behavioral couples therapy for alcoholism and drug abuse: Where we've been, where we are, and where we're going. *Journal of Cognitive Psychotherapy* 19(3):229-246.

Fann, J. R., T. Hart, and K. G. Schomer. 2009. Treatment for depression after traumatic brain injury: A systematic review. *Journal of Neurotrauma* 26(12):2383-2402.

FDA (Food and Drug Administration). 2012. *Guidance for Industry: Suicidal Ideation and Behavior: Prospective Assessment of Occurrence in Clinical Trials.* http://www.fda.gov/downloads/Drugs/.../Guidances/UCM225130.pdf (accessed November 11, 2012).

Fleischmann, A., J. M. Bertolote, D. Wasserman, D. De Leo, J. Bolhari, N. J. Botega, D. De Silva, M. Phillips, L. Vijayakumar, A. Varnik, L. Schlebusch, and H. T. T. Thanh. 2008. Effectiveness of brief intervention and contact for suicide attempters: A randomized controlled trial in five countries. *Bulletin of the World Health Organization* 86(9):703-709.

Foa, E. B., T. M. Keane, J. Friedman, and J. A. Cohen. 2009. *Effective Treatments for PTSD: Practice Guidelines from the International Society for Traumatic Stress Studies.* 2nd ed. New York: Guilford Publications.

Ford, A. C., and P. O. Vandvik. 2012. Irritable bowel syndrome. *Clinical Evidence.* 01:410.

Ford, A. C., N. J. Talley, P. S. Schoenfeld, E. M. Quigley, and P. Moayyedi. 2009. Efficacy of antidepressants and psychological therapies in irritable bowel syndrome: Systematic review and meta-analysis. *Gut* 58(3):367-378.

Ford, J. D., K. A. Campbell, D. Storzbach, L. M. Binder, W. K. Anger, and D. S. Rohlman. 2001. Posttraumatic stress symptomatology is associated with unexplained illness attributed to Persian Gulf War military service. *Psychosomatic Medicine* 63(5):842-849.

Friedman, M. J., P. A. Resick, R. A. Bryant, and C. R. Brewin. 2011. Considering PTSD for DSM-5. *Depression and Anxiety* 28(9):750-769.

Friedman, R., V. Li, and D. Mehrotra. 2003. Treating pain patients at risk: Evaluation of a screening tool in opioid-treated pain patients with and without addiction. *Pain Medicine* 4(2):182-185.

Gill, A., R. Womack, and S. Safranek. 2010. Does exercise alleviate symptoms of depression? *Journal of Family Practice* 59(9):530-531.

Glaser, R., and J. K. Kiecolt-Glaser. 1998. Stress-associated immune modulation: Relevance to viral infections and chronic fatigue syndrome. *American Journal of Medicine* 105(3A):35S-42S.

Gordon, W. A., L. Haddad, M. Brown, M. R. Hibbard, and M. Sliwinski. 2000. The sensitivity and specificity and self-reported symptoms in people with traumatic brain injury. *Brain Injury* 14(1):21-33.

Grover, M., and D. A. Drossman. 2009. Psychopharmacologic and behavioral treatments for functional gastrointestinal disorders. *Gastroenterology Endoscopy Clinics of North America* 19(1):151-170.

Haney, E. M., M. E. O'Neil, S. Carson, A. Low, K. Peterson, L. M. Denneson, C. Oleksiewicz, and D. Kansagara. 2012. *Suicide Risk Factors and Risk Assessment Tools: A Systematic Review.* Department of Veterans Affairs—Evidence-Based Synthesis Program. http://www.hsrd.research.va.gov/publications/esp/suicide-risk.pdf (accessed November 11, 2012).

Harber, V. J., and J. R. Sutton. 1984. Endorphins and exercise. *Sports Medicine* 1(2):154-171. http://www.ncbi.nlm.nih.gov/pubmed/6091217 (accessed November 11, 2012).

Hasin, D., and H. Katz. 2007. Somatoform and substance use disorders. *Psychosomatic Medicine* 69(9):870-875.

Hauser, W., K. Bernardy, B. Arnold, M. Offenbacher, and M. Schiltenwolf. 2009. Efficacy of multicomponent treatment in fibromyalgia syndrome: A meta-analysis of randomized controlled clinical trials. *Arthritis & Rheumatism-Arthritis Care & Research* 61(2):216-224.

Hauser, W., F. Petzke, N. Uceyler, and C. Sommer. 2011. Comparative efficacy and acceptability of amitriptyline, duloxetine and milnacipran in fibromyalgia syndrome: A systematic review with meta-analysis. *Rheumatology* 50(3):532-543.

Hays, R. D., K. B. Wells, C. D. Sherbourne, W. Rogers, and K. Spritzer. 1995. Functioning and well-being outcomes of patients with depression compared with chronic general medical illnesses. *Archives of General Psychiatry* 52(1):11-19.

Helmick, K. 2010. Cognitive rehabilitation for military personnel with mild traumatic brain injury and chronic post-concussional disorder: Results of April 2009 Consensus Conference. *Neurorehabilitation* 26(3):239-255.

Hibbard, M. R., S. Uysal, K. Kepler, J. Bogdany, and J. Silver. 1998. Axis I psychopathology in individuals with traumatic brain injury. *Journal of Head Trauma Rehabilitation* 13(4):24-39.

Hinton, D. E., and R. Lewis-Fernandez. 2011. The cross-cultural validity of posttraumatic stress disorder: Implications for DSM-5. *Depression and Anxiety* 28(9):783-801.

Ilgen, M. A., A. S. B. Bohnert, R. V. Ignacio, J. F. McCarthy, M. M. Valenstein, H. M. Kim, and F. C. Blow. 2010. Psychiatric diagnoses and risk of suicide in veterans. *Archives of General Psychiatry* 67(11):1152-1158.

IOM (Institute of Medicine). 2006. *Gulf War and Health, Volume 4: Health Effects of Serving in the Gulf War.* Washington, DC: The National Academies Press.

IOM. 2007. *Treatment of PTSD: An Assessment of the Evidence.* Washington, DC: The National Academies Press.

IOM. 2010. *Gulf War and Health, Volume 8: Update of Health Effects of Serving in the Gulf War.* Washington, DC: The National Academies Press.

IOM. 2011a. *Cognitive Rehabilitation Therapy for Traumatic Brain Injury: Evaluating the Evidence.* Washington, DC: The National Academies Press.

IOM. 2011b. *Relieving Pain in America: A Blue Print for Transforming Prevention, Care, Education, and Research.* Washington, DC: The National Academies Press.

IOM. 2012. *Treatment for Posttraumatic Stress Disorder in Military and Veteran Populations: Initial Assessment.* Washington, DC: The National Academies Press.

Jackson, J. L., P. G. O'Malley, G. Tomkins, E. Balden, J. Santoro, and K. Kroenke. 2000. Treatment of functional gastrointestinal disorders with antidepressant medications: A meta-analysis. *American Journal of Medicine* 108(1):65-72.

Jacobs, D. G., and M. L. Brewer. 2006. Application of the APA Practice Guidelines on suicide to clinical practice. *CNS Spectrums* 11(6):447-454.

Jason, L. A., N. Porter, J. Hunnell, A. Brown, A. Rademaker, and J. A. Richman. 2011. A natural history study of chronic fatigue syndrome. *Rehabilitation Psychology* 56(1):32-42.

Joiner, T. E., and K. A. Van Orden. 2008. The interpersonal-psychological theory of suicidal behavior indicates specific and crucial psychotherapeutic targets. *International Journal of Cognitive Therapy* 1(1):80-89.

Katon, W. J., and E. A. Walker. 1998. Medically unexplained symptoms in primary care. *Journal of Clinical Psychiatry* 59(Suppl 20):15-21.

Katsamanis, M., P. M. Lehrer, J. I. Escobar, M. A. Gara, A. Kotay, and R. Liu. 2011. Psychophysiologic treatment for patients with medically unexplained symptoms: A randomized controlled trial. *Psychosomatics* 52(3):218-229.

Krilov, L. R., M. Fisher, S. B. Friedman, D. Reitman, and F. S. Mandel. 1998. Course and outcome of chronic fatigue in children and adolescents. *Pediatrics* 102(2):360-366.

Kroenke, K., R. L. Spitzer, and J. B. W. Williams. 2001. The PHQ-9: Validity of a brief depression severity measure. *Journal of General Internal Medicine* 16(9):606-613.

Kroenke, K., N. Messina, I. Benattia, J. Graepel, and J. Musgnung. 2006. Venlafaxine extended release in the short-term treatment of depressed and anxious primary care patients with multisomatoform disorder. *Journal of Clinical Psychiatry* 67(1):72-80.

Lackner, J. M., J. Jaccard, S. S. Krasner, L. A. Katz, G. D. Gudleski, and K. Holroyd. 2008. Self-administered cognitive behavior therapy for moderate to severe irritable bowel syndrome: Clinical efficacy, tolerability, feasibility. *Clinical Gastroenterology and Hepatology* 6(8):899-906.

Lancaster, T., and L. F. Stead. 2005. Individual behavioural counselling for smoking cessation. *Cochrane Database of Systematic Reviews* Issue 2. Art. No.: CD001292.

Lawrence, R. C., D. T. Felson, C. G. Helmick, L. M. Arnold, H. Choi, R. A. Deyo, S. Gabriel, R. Hirsch, M. C. Hochberg, G. G. Hunder, J. M. Jordan, J. N. Katz, H. M. Kremers, and F. Wolfe. 2008. Estimates of the prevalence of arthritis and other rheumatic conditions in the United States. *Arthritis and Rheumatism* 58(1):26-35.

Lee, C., J. Smith, M. Sprengel, C. Crawford, D. Wallerstedt, R. Welton, A. York, A. Duncan, and W. B. Jonas. 2012. An assessment of the effectiveness of acupuncture for the trauma spectrum response: Results of a rapid evidence assessment of the literature (REAL). *BMC Complementary and Alternative Medicine* 12(Suppl 1).

Lesbros-Pantoflickova, D., P. Michetti, M. Fried, C. Beglinger, and A. L. Blum. 2004. Meta-analysis: The treatment of irritable bowel syndrome. *Alimentary Pharmacology & Therapeutics* 20(11-12):1253-1269.

Levy, R. L., K. W. Olden, B. D. Naliboff, L. A. Bradley, C. Francisconi, D. A. Drossman, and F. Creed. 2006. Psychosocial aspects of the functional gastrointestinal disorders. *Gastroenterology* 130(5):1447-1458.

Lew, H. L., J. D. Otis, C. Tun, R. D. Kerns, M. E. Clark, and D. X. Cifu. 2009. Prevalence of chronic pain, posttraumatic stress disorder, and persistent postconcussive symptoms in OIF/OEF veterans: Polytrauma clinical triad. *Journal of Rehabilitation Research and Development* 46(6):697-702.

Lindfors, P., P. Unge, P. Arvidsson, H. Nyhlin, E. Bjornsson, H. Abrahamsson, and M. Simren. 2012. Effects of gut-directed hypnotherapy on IBS in different clinical settings: Results from two randomized, controlled trials. *American Journal of Gastroenterology* 107(2):276-285.

Longstreth, G. F., W. G. Thompson, W. D. Chey, L. A. Houghton, F. Mearin, and R. C. Spiller. 2006. Functional bowel disorders. *Gastroenterology* 130(5):1480-1491.

Luoma, J. B., C. E. Martin, and J. L. Pearson. 2002. Contact with mental health and primary care providers before suicide: A review of the evidence. *American Journal of Psychiatry* 159(6):909-916.

Manheimer, E., A. White, B. Berman, K. Forys, and E. Ernst. 2005. Acupuncture for low back pain. *Annals of Internal Medicine* 143(9):695-695.

Maquet, D., C. Demoulin, and J. M. Crielaard. 2006. Chronic fatigue syndrome: A systematic review. *Annales de Readaptation et de Médecine Physique* 49(6):337-347, 418-327.

Maquet, D., C. Demoulin, J. L. Croisier, and J. M. Crielaard. 2007. Benefits of physical training in fibromyalgia and related syndromes. *Annales de Readaptation et de Médecine Physique* 50(6):356-362, 363-368.

Mayo Clinic Staff. 2011. *Chronic Fatigue Syndrome: Treatments and Drugs*. http://www.mayoclinic.com/health/chronic-fatigue-syndrome/ds00395/dsection=treatments-and-drugs (accessed November 11, 2012).

McWhinney, I. R., R. M. Epstein, and T. R. Freeman. 2001. Rethinking somatization. *Advances in Mind Body Medicine* 17(4):235-239.

Menon, D. K., K. Schwab, D. W. Wright, and A. I. Maas. 2010. Position statement: Definition of traumatic brain injury. *Archives of Physical Medicine and Rehabilitation* 91(11):1637-1640.

Mertz, H., R. Fass, A. Kodner, F. Yan-Go, S. Fullerton, and E. A. Mayer. 1998. Effect of amitryptiline on symptoms, sleep, and visceral perception in patients with functional dyspepsia. *American Journal of Gastroenterology* 93(2):160-165.

Moldofsky, H. 1993. Fibromyalgia, sleep disorder and chronic fatigue syndrome. *Ciba Foundation Symposia* 173:262-279.

Moore, R. A., S. Straube, P. J. Wiffen, S. Derry, and H. J. McQuay. 2009. Pregabalin for acute and chronic pain in adults. *Cochrane Database of Systematic Reviews* Issue 3. Art. No.: CD007076.

Moore, R. A., P. J. Wiffen, S. Derry, and H. J. McQuay. 2011. Gabapentin for chronic neuropathic pain and fibromyalgia in adults. *Cochrane Database of Systematic Reviews* Issue 3. Art. No.: CD007938.

Motto, J. A., and A. G. Bostrom. 2001. A randomized controlled trial of postcrisis suicide prevention. *Psychiatric Services* 52(6):828-833.

National Collaborating Centre for Mental Health. 2004. *Self Harm: The Short-Term Physical and Psychological Management and Secondary Prevention of Self-Harm in Primary and Secondary Care*. London: National Institute for Health and Clinical Excellence. http://www.nice.org.uk/nicemedia/pdf/CG016NICEguideline.pdf (accessed November 11, 2012).

National Collaborating Centre for Mental Health. 2005. *Post-Traumatic Stress Disorder (PTSD): The Management of PTSD In Adults and Children in Primary and Secondary Care.* London: National Institute of Health and Clinical Excellence. http://www.nice.org.uk/nicemedia/live/10966/29769/29769.pdf (accessed November 11, 2012).

National Collaborating Centre for Mental Health. 2009a. *Depression in Adults with a Chronic Physical Health Problem.* London: National Institute of Health and Clinical Excellence. http://www.nice.org.uk/CG91 (accessed November 11, 2012).

National Collaborating Centre for Mental Health. 2009b. *Depression: The Treatment and Management of Depression in Adults.* London: National Institute of Health and Clinical Excellence. http://www.nice.org.uk/nicemedia/pdf/Depression_Update_FULL_GUIDELINE.pdf (accessed November 11, 2012).

National Collaborating Centre for Mental Health. 2011. *Alcohol Dependence and Harmful Alcohol Use.* London: National Institute for Health and Clinical Excellence. http://guidance.nice.org.uk/CG115 (accessed November 11, 2012).

National Collaborating Centre for Mental Health and National Collaborating Centre for Primary Care. 2011a. *Generalized Anxiety Disorder and Panic Disorder (With Or Without Agoraphobia) in Adults: Management in Primary, Secondary and Community Care.* London: National Institute for Health and Clinical Excellence. http://www.nice.org.uk/nicemedia/live/13314/52599/52599.pdf (accessed November 11, 2012).

National Collaborating Centre for Mental Health and National Collaborating Centre for Primary Care. 2011b. *Longer-term Care and Treatment of Self-harm.* London: National Institute for Health and Clinical Excellence. http://www.nice.org.uk/nicemedia/live/13619/57175/57175.pdf (accessed November 11, 2012).

National Collaborating Centre for Primary Care. 2007. *Chronic Fatigue Syndrome/Myalgic Encephalomyelitis (or Encephalopathy): Diagnosis and Management of CFS/ME in Adults and Children.* London: National Institute for Health and Clinical Excellence. http://www.nice.org.uk/nicemedia/live/11824/36193/36193.pdf (accessed November 11, 2012).

NIDA (National Institute on Drug Abuse). 2009. *Principles of Drug Addiction Treatment: A Research-based Guide.* Bethesda, MD: National Institutes of Health. http://www.drugabuse.gov/sites/default/files/podat_0.pdf (accessed November 11, 2012).

Nieuwsma, J. A., R. B. Trivedi, J. McDuffie, I. Kronish, D. Benjamin, and J. W. Williams. 2012. Brief psychotherapy for depression: A systematic review and meta-analysis. *International Journal of Psychiatry in Medicine* 43(2):129-151.

NIH (National Institutes of Health). 2012a. *Generalized Anxiety Disorders Among Adults.* http://www.nimh.nih.gov/statistics/1GAD_ADULT.shtml (accessed September 27, 2012).

NIH. 2012b. *The Numbers Count: Mental Disorders in America.* http://www.nimh.nih.gov/health/publications/the-numbers-count-mental-disorders-in-america/index.shtml (accessed September 27, 2012).

Nishishinya, B., G. Urrutia, B. Walitt, A. Rodriguez, X. Bonfill, C. Alegre, and G. Darko. 2008. Amitriptyline in the treatment of fibromyalgia: A systematic review of its efficacy. *Rheumatology* 47(12):1741-1746.

Nuesch, E., W. Hauser, K. Bernardy, J. Barth, and P. Juni. 2012. Comparative efficacy of pharmacological and non-pharmacological interventions in fibromyalgia syndrome: Network meta-analysis. *Annals of the Rheumatic Diseases* Epub.

Olatunji, B. O., J. M. Cisler, and D. F. Tolin. 2010. A meta-analysis of the influence of comorbidity on treatment outcome in the anxiety disorders. *Clinical Psychology Review* 30(6):642-654.

Palsson, O. S., and W. E. Whitehead. 2002. The growing case for hypnosis as adjunctive therapy for functional gastrointestinal disorders. *Gastroenterology* 123(6):2132-2135.

Pan, Y. J., M. B. Lee, H. C. Chiang, and S. C. Liao. 2009. The recognition of diagnosable psychiatric disorders in suicide cases' last medical contacts. *General Hospital Psychiatry* 31(2):181-184.

Park, S., M. J. Cho, S. Seong, S. Y. Shin, J. Sohn, B. J. Hahm, and J. P. Hong. 2012. Psychiatric morbidities, sleep disturbances, suicidality, and quality-of-life in a community population with medically unexplained pain in Korea. *Psychiatric Research* 198(3):509-515.

Posner, K., G. K. Brown, B. Stanley, D. A. Brent, K. V. Yershova, M. A. Oquendo, G. W. Currier, G. A. Melvin, L. Greenhill, S. Shen, and J. J. Mann. 2011. The Columbia-Suicide Severity Rating Scale: Initial validity and internal consistency findings from three multisite studies with adolescents and adults. *American Journal of Psychiatry* 168(12):1266-1277.

Prins, A., P. Ouimette, R. Kimerling, R. P. Cameron, D. S. Hugelshofer, J. Shaw-Hegwer, A. Thrailkill, F. D. Gusman, and J. I. Sheikh. 2003. The primary care PTSD screen (PC-PTSD): Development and operating characteristics. *Primary Care Psychiatry* 9(1):9-14.

Quigley, K. S., L. M. McAndrew, L. Almeida, E. A. D'Andrea, C. C. Engel, H. Hamtil, and A. J. Ackerman. 2012. Prevalence of environmental and other military exposure concerns in Operation Enduring Freedom and Operation Iraqi Freedom veterans. *Journal of Occupational & Environmental Medicine* 54(6):659-664.

Rainville, P., R. K. Hofbauer, T. Paus, G. H. Duncan, M. C. Bushnell, and D. D. Price. 1999. Cerebral mechanisms of hypnotic induction and suggestion. *Journal of Cognitive Neuroscience* 11(1):110-125.

Reeves, W. C., J. F. Jones, E. Maloney, C. Heim, D. C. Hoaglin, R. S. Boneva, M. Morrissey, and R. Devlin. 2007. Prevalence of chronic fatigue syndrome in metropolitan, urban and rural Georgia. *Population Health Metrics* 5(5).

Regier, D. A., M. E. Farmer, D. S. Rae, B. Z. Locke, S. J. Keith, L. L. Judd, and F. K. Goodwin. 1990. Comorbidity of mental-disorders with alcohol and other drug-abuse: Results from the Epidemiologic Catchment-Area (ECA) Study. *Journal of the American Medical Association* 264(19):2511-2518.

Rimer, J., K. Dwan, D. A. Lawlor, C. A. Greig, M. McMurdo, W. Morley, and G. E. Mead. 2012. Exercise for depression. *Cochrane Database of Systematic Reviews* Issue 7. Art. No.: CD004366.

Russell, I. J., M. Kamin, R. M. Bennett, T. J. Schnitzer, J. A. Green, and W. A. Katz. 2000. Efficacy of tramadol in treatment of pain in fibromyalgia. *Journal of Clinical Rheumatology* 6(5):250-257.

Schutte-Rodin, S., L. Broch, D. Buysse, C. Dorsey, and M. Satei. 2008. Clinical guideline for the evaluation and management of chronic insomnia in adults. *Journal of Clinical Sleep Medicine* 4(5):487-504.

Sheldon, L. K., S. Swanson, A. Dolce, K. Marsh, and J. Summers. 2008. Putting evidence into practice: Evidence-based interventions for anxiety. *Clinical Journal of Oncology Nursing* 12(5):789-797.

Shorter, E. 1993. *Paralysis to Fatigue: A History of Psychosomatic Illness in the Modern Era.* New York, NY: The Free Press.

Siler, A. C., H. Gardner, K. Yanit, T. Cushman, and M. McDonagh. 2011. Systematic review of the comparative effectiveness of antiepileptic drugs for fibromyalgia. *Journal of Pain* 12(4):407-415.

Sledjeski, E. M., B. Speisman, and L. C. Dierker. 2008. Does number of lifetime traumas explain the relationship between PTSD and chronic medical conditions? Answers from The National Comorbidity Survey Replication (NCS-R). *Journal of Behavioral Medicine* 31(4):341-349.

Soo, C., R. L. Tate, and A. Lane-Brown. 2011. A systematic review of Acceptance and Commitment Therapy (ACT) for managing anxiety: Applicability for people with acquired brain injury? *Brain Impairment* 12(1):54-70.

Stead, L. F., and T. Lancaster. 2008. Intervention review: Group behaviour therapy programmes for smoking cessation. *The Cochrane Library* Issue 2. Art. No.: CD001007.

Storzbach, D., K. A. Campbell, L. M. Binder, L. McCauley, W. K. Anger, D. S. Rohlman, C. A. Kovera, and C. Portland Env Hazards Res. 2000. Psychological differences between veterans with and without Gulf War unexplained symptoms. *Psychosomatic Medicine* 62(5):726-735.

Sultan, A., H. Gaskell, S. Derry, and R. A. Moore. 2008. Duloxetine for painful diabetic neuropathy and fibromyalgia pain: Systematic review of randomised trials. *BMC Neurology* 8:29.

Tack, J., N. J. Talley, M. Camilleri, G. Holtmann, P. Hu, J. R. Malagelada, and V. Stanghellini. 2006. Functional gastroduodenal disorders. *Gastroenterology* 130(5):1466-1479.

Thiwan, S. M., and D. A. Drossman. 2006. Treatment of functional GI disorders with psychotropic medicines: A review of evidence with a practical approach. *Gastroenterology and Hepatology* 2(9):678-688.

Tzellos, T. G., K. A. Toulis, D. G. Goulis, G. Papazisis, V. A. Zampeli, A. Vakfari, and D. Kouvelas. 2010. Gabapentin and pregabalin in the treatment of fibromyalgia: A systematic review and a meta-analysis. *Journal of Clinical Pharmacy and Therapeutics* 35(6):639-656.

Uceyler, N., W. Hauser, and C. Sommer. 2008. A systematic review on the effectiveness of treatment with antidepressants in fibromyalgia syndrome. *Arthritis & Rheumatism* 59(9):1279-1298.

US Army. 2010. *Army Health Promotion/Risk Reduction/Suicide Prevention Report 2010.* Washington, DC. http://www.apd.army.mil/pdffiles/p600_24.pdf (accessed November 11, 2012).

VA (Department of Veterans Affairs) and DOD (Department of Defense). 2009a. *Clinical Practice Guideline: Management of Concussion/Mild Traumatic Brain Injury.* http://www.healthquality.va.gov/mtbi/concussion_mtbi_full_1_0.pdf (accessed November 11, 2012).

VA and DOD. 2009b. *Clinical Practice Guideline: Management of Major Depressive Disorder* (MDD). http://www.healthquality.va.gov/MDD_FULL_3c.pdf (accessed November 11, 2012).

VA and DOD. 2009c. *VA/DOD Essentials for Depression Screening and Assessment in Primary Care.* http://www.healthquality.va.gov/mdd/MDDTool1VADoDEssentialsQuadFoldFinal HiRes.pdf (accessed November 11, 2012).

VA and DOD. 2010a. *Clinical Practice Guideline for Management of Post-Traumatic Stress.* http://www.healthquality.va.gov/ptsd/PTSD-FULL-2010a.pdf (accessed November 11, 2012).

VA and DOD. 2010b. *Clinical Practice Guideline: Management of Opioid Therapy for Chronic Pain.* http://www.healthquality.va.gov/COT_312_Full-er.pdf (accessed November 11, 2012).

Van Kerkhoven, L. A. S., R. J. F. Laheij, N. Aparicio, W. A. De Boer, S. Van Den Hazel, A. Tan, B. J. M. Witteman, and J. Jansen. 2008. Effect of the antidepressant venlafaxine in functional dyspepsia: A randomized, double-blind, placebo-controlled trial. *Clinical Gastroenterology and Hepatology* 6(7):746-752.

Vickers, A. J. 2012. Acupuncture for chronic pain: Individual patient data meta-analysis. *Archives of Internal Medicine.*

Walker, R. L., M. E. Clark, and S. H. Sanders. 2010. The "postdeployment multi-symptom disorder": An emerging syndrome in need of a new treatment paradigm. *Psychological Services* 7(3):136-147.

Watson, D. 2005. Rethinking the mood and anxiety disorders: A quantitative hierarchical model for DSM-V. *Journal of Abnormal Psychology* 114 (4):522-536.

WFMH (World Federation for Mental Health). 2010. *Mental Health and Chronic Physical Illnesses: The Need for Continued and Integrated Care.* http://www.wfmh.org/2010DOCS/WMHDAY2010.pdf (accessed November 11, 2012)

WGO (World Gastroenterology Organisation). 2009. *Irritable Bowel Syndrome: A Global Perspective.* Munich.

Whitehead, W. E. 2006. Hypnosis for irritable bowel syndrome: The empirical evidence of therapeutic effects. *International Journal of Clinical and Experimental Hypnosis* 54(1):7-20.

Whorwell, P. J., A. Prior, and S. M. Colgan. 1987. Hypnotherapy in severe irritable bowel syndrome: Further experience. *Gut* 28(4):423-425.

Wilson, S., T. Maddison, L. Roberts, S. Greenfield, S. Singh, and I. B. S. R. G. Birmingham. 2006. Systematic review: The effectiveness of hypnotherapy in the management of irritable bowel syndrome. *Alimentary Pharmacology & Therapeutics* 24(5):769-780.

Wolfe, F., H. A. Smythe, M. B. Yunus, R. M. Bennett, C. Bombardier, D. L. Goldenberg, P. Tugwell, S. M. Campbell, M. Abeles, P. Clark, A. G. Fam, S. J. Farber, J. J. Fiechtner, C. M. Franklin, R. A. Gatter, D. Hamaty, J. Lessard, A. S. Lichtbroun, A. T. Masi, G. A. McCain, W. J. Reynolds, T. J. Romano, I. J. Russell, and R. P. Sheon. 1990. The American College of Rheumatology 1990 criteria for the classification of fibromyalgia: Report of the Multicenter Criteria Committee. *Arthritis and Rheumatism* 33(2):160-172.

Wolfe, F., D. J. Clauw, M. A. Fitzcharles, D. L. Goldenberg, R. S. Katz, P. Mease, A. S. Russell, I. J. Russell, J. B. Winfield, and M. B. Yunus. 2010. The American College of Rheumatology preliminary diagnostic criteria for fibromyalgia and measurement of symptom severity. *Arthritis Care and Research* 62(5):600-610.

6

Patient-Centered Care of Veterans Who Have Chronic Multisymptom Illness

This chapter presents a patient-centered approach to the management of care of veterans who have chronic multisymptom illness (CMI). It discusses patient–clinician interactions with a focus on improving communication. It also considers how the new information and communication technologies could be harnessed to improve care.

CLINICIAN TRAINING, PRACTICE BEHAVIORS, AND CHRONIC MULTISYMPTOM ILLNESS

The treatment of veterans for CMI requires a multipronged approach. A major determinant of success in practice behaviors is the training of clinicians, who can include physicians (primary care physicians and specialists), physician assistants, nurses, mental health therapists, and physical rehabilitation therapists, in the particulars of how patients who have CMI are best managed. Training (investment in human capital) of clinical teams has been found to be a critical factor in the adoption and maintenance of innovations (Smits et al., 2008). In many cases, physicians are unprepared for or not trained in managing the care of patients who have CMI, or the systems in which they practice do not enable them to address how to work with such patients. (Practice and systems issues are addressed in Chapter 7.) Although it is generally recognized that training physicians and other clinicians in caring for people who have CMI may matter, there have been few systematic studies, including randomized controlled trials (RCTs); however, there have been several qualitative or observational studies whose results offer some useful insights into the value of training clinicians about CMI.

Training of clinicians about the challenges faced by patients who are suffering from medically unexplained symptoms (referred to as CMI in this report) appears to have changed their attitudes toward the patients (Fazekas et al., 2009). In one study, although physicians recognized the challenges and suffering of veterans who had medically unexplained symptoms, they were wary of the difficulty in treating the patients (Aiarzaguena et al., 2009). Even participation in a "brief exposure," such as a seminar, may make clinicians more receptive to and sympathetic toward patients who have medically unexplained symptoms, according to a study of medical students (Friedberg et al., 2008).

In one RCT, training of physicians in communication skills and in treating patients who have CMI resulted in greater patient satisfaction (Frostholm et al., 2005). Patients who had more uncertainty and negative emotions (feeling worried, depressed, helpless, afraid, or hopeless) about their health problems were less satisfied with the consultations with their physicians.

Evidence on the effectiveness of current methods of teaching clinicians how to communicate is sparse. In a recent comprehensive review of physician communication, Christianson et al. (2012) described the complexities of improving physician–patient communication. They documented that although training in communication skills is an important component of improving patient care, such training alone is insufficient. Additional factors need to be addressed, including

- Patient characteristics, such as sex, ethnicity, age, physical appearance, education or language and literacy, and the presence of a terminal illnesses or chronic condition (such as CMI).
- Practice characteristics, such as physical surroundings that are crowded and noisy, the availability of "decision aids" or electronic health records, and in-office laboratories and imaging equipment.
- Environmental characteristics, which may be financial (for example, fee-for-service reimbursement, pressure to see more patients in the practice day leading to reduced visit length, or increasing payment by overuse or misuse of procedures and laboratory studies) and the need to use evidence-based treatment guidelines, potentially creating time-management problems for physician practices (Ostbye et al., 2005).

Christianson et al. (2012) stated that "possible interventions to improve physician communication . . . typically focus exclusively on the role of physician characteristics and give relatively little attention to mediating factors related to practice setting or patient characteristics. By doing so, they risk . . . overlook[ing] potentially fruitful interventions to improve communication that could be directed at altering mediating factors."

Clinician training involving a comprehensive approach that combines pharmacologic therapy with biopsychosocial, cognitive behavioral, and case-management skills training or that emphasizes specific reattribution training (see next paragraph) has been found to be effective in managing patients who have CMI. Studies that provided comprehensive training for clinicians tended to show substantial benefit in physical functioning and mental health in patients even after 6–24 months of follow-up. For example, training clinicians to use a multifaceted intervention combining appropriate medications based on symptoms, cognitive behavioral therapy (CBT), and a specific patient-centered method proved beneficial in several studies (Smith and Dwamena, 2007; Smith et al., 2003, 2006, 2009). Similarly, Margalit and El-Ad (2008) demonstrated decreased hospital days and emergency room visits at both the 1-year and 2-year points after CBT, medication, and other therapies were administered by clinicians with expertise in treating patients who have CMI. Improvement in physical functioning and mental health was observed in patients who have CMI 12 months after the use of effective case management plans developed by an expert group of clinicians (Pols and Battersby, 2008). Finally, a collaborative-care model with CBT and side-by-side psychiatric consultation with the primary care clinician showed improvement in the severity of symptoms and in social functioning and decreased health care use after 6 months (Van Der Feltz-Cornelis et al., 2006). In that study, the primary care clinicians were trained in case management and CBT.

Reattribution training involves skills in empathizing with patients regarding their physical complaints and helping them to connect their physical symptoms with their emotions and psychosocial circumstances. Studies based on reattribution training have had mixed results. There were mild decreases in physical symptoms and pain (Aiarzaguena et al., 2007; Larisch et al., 2004) and some improvement in patient satisfaction with physician–patient communication (Morriss et al., 2007). However, two studies that examined the impact of "the extended reattribution and management" model in which clinicians received training in biopsychosocial history taking and management strategies in addition to reattribution training showed no long-term benefits (Rosendal et al., 2007; Toft et al., 2010), although one of them (Toft et al., 2010) showed mild benefits of improved physical functioning at 3 months.

The effectiveness of another form of clinician training, consultation with a mental health professional with or without consultation letters, also has been studied. Consultation letters educate the referring clinician about the chronic nature of the symptoms and suggest treatment strategies for the care team to use that are based on frequency of follow-up visits and psychosocial models rather than high-cost testing and procedures. Consultations with mental health experts did not appear to be effective on their own (Rasmussen et al., 2006; Schilte et al., 2001). Rasmussen et al. (2006) examined the benefits of a reflecting interview for their patients who had CMI. The patients were interviewed about their diagnosis, their condition, and optimal ways of treating for their symptoms. Although there were no differences in health scores (SF-12) between the treatment and control groups after 6 or 12 months, there were significant reductions in health care costs in the intervention group after 1 year. Similarly, Shilte et al. (2001) studied the impact of disclosure of emotionality in patients who had medically unexplained symptoms. Patients in the intervention group of this RCT were asked to disclose important events in their lives. They were psychiatrically screened and were asked to keep a diary of their thoughts, emotions, and physical complaints. There was no significant improvement in the physical or psychologic health of the intervention group after the 2-year study period.

IMPROVING COMMUNICATION SKILLS AND THE PATIENT–CLINICIAN RELATIONSHIP

The information acquired thus far regarding the perceptions and possible experiences of veterans who have multisymptom or other functional syndromes and are returning from deployment makes it evident that treatment must begin with establishing an effective patient–clinician relationship. That premise is supported by results of several studies that show that good communication skills and an effective patient–clinician relationship can lead to improved patient satisfaction, better disclosure of important information, greater adherence to treatment, reduced emotional distress, improved physiologic measures, and better overall clinical outcomes (Anderson et al., 2008; Frostholm et al., 2005; Hall et al., 2002; Roter and Hall, 1989, 1992; Roter et al., 1995). Conversely, ineffective communication skills and a poor patient–clinician relationship are associated with low patient satisfaction and even an increase in malpractice claims (Levinson et al., 1997).

The basic practices of any good clinician communication in patient encounters were thoroughly documented in what has been called the Kalamazoo Consensus Statement of 1999 (Makoul, 2001). They include allowing the patient to complete his or her "opening statement"; eliciting concerns and establishing a rapport with the patient; using a combination of open-ended and closed-ended questions to gather and clarify information and different listening techniques to solicit information; identifying and responding to the patient's personal situation, beliefs, and values; using language that the patient can understand to explain diagnoses and treatment plans; checking for patient understanding; encouraging the patient to participate in decisions and exploring the patient's willingness and ability to follow care plans; asking for other concerns that the patient might have;

and discussing follow-up activities expected of the patient before closing the visit (Makoul, 2001, p. 391).

Patient Perceptions Regarding the Patient–Clinician Relationship and Chronic Multisymptom Illness

On the basis of clinical studies, patient presentations to the committee,[1] and a social media analysis commissioned by the committee (Furey, 2012), the committee made several observations to be considered in developing recommendations to improve the relationship between clinicians and patients who have CMI:

- Many patients who have CMI do not believe that they are receiving proper care.
- Patients believe that clinicians focus on diagnosis and on treatment for symptoms rather than on seeking out the underlying condition. In one research study, clinicians did less exploration of symptoms and validation when seeing CMI patients than when seeing patients who had clear-cut symptoms, such as esophageal reflux disease (Epstein et al., 2006).
- Patients feel that their clinicians do not understand or believe their symptoms, and they desperately want to be believed. They fear that clinicians believe that "it's all in your mind," and they feel isolated almost as "medical orphans" (Nettleton et al., 2005). Although it is unlikely that clinicians have communicated such perspectives directly, there are sufficient patient commentaries to suggest that it is occurring indirectly either through faulty communication and nonverbal behaviors or through dialogue that communicates mixed messages or clinician uncertainty (olde Hartman et al., 2009).
- Patients do not feel that their clinicians fully consider the whole person or explore his or her life experience. They would like clinicians to understand the effects of CMI on work, social, and family life, understand the patient's expectations and beliefs, and recognize the influence of ethnic or sociocultural norms. Because patients who have CMI may not directly state the full effects of their disorder, the clinician might tend to ignore or minimize their life experience and focus more clinically in dealing with the symptoms (Kappen and van Dulmen, 2008; Ring et al., 2004; Salmon et al., 2007).

---

[1]Comments were made to the committee during public sessions held on December 12, 2011, and February 29, 2012. The committee also received written comments from members of the public, which can be obtained by contacting the National Academies Public Access Records Office (see http://www8.nationalacademies.org/cp/projectview.aspx?key=49405).

- There appears to be a discrepancy between patients' and their peers' beliefs and their clinicians' beliefs about the cause of and possible treatments for the condition. That gap in perceptions must be reconciled to improve the outcome. A patient's beliefs can influence the severity of the symptoms and daily functioning (Hunt et al., 2004).
- Many patients are seeking alternative treatments because they are dissatisfied with the type of care received from their health care clinicians.
- Patients want to participate in decision making regarding options for their treatment. Health literacy may affect the transfer of information that enables decision making.
- Family members are affected by the multisymptom illness and need to be involved in the patient's education and possibly in care decisions.
- Patients who feel uncertain about their illness and are involved negatively with their health problems (that is, worried, depressed, helpless, and hopeless) tend to be dissatisfied with their care, as the committee has seen in patients with CMI and their clinicians (Frostholm et al., 2005). However, patients are more satisfied with clinicians who are trained in good communication (Frostholm et al., 2005). That finding highlights the value of learning good communication techniques.

Factors Related to Good Patient–Clinician Interactions

The committee believes that an effective patient–clinician relationship is the foundation of treatment for CMI and is necessary if patients who have CMI are to derive maximum benefit from any specific treatment. Guidelines developed by expert clinicians and educators and established by consensus are used to teach clinicians good communication techniques (Chang and Drossman, 2002; Drossman, 1999; Fortin et al., 2012; Lipkin et al., 1995; Morgan and Engel, 1969; Roter and Hall, 1992). Those guidelines, along with the work of other researchers, provide the basis for the committee's discussion below on improving the patient–clinician relationship.

Many of the strategies described below are similar to the concept of motivational interviewing (MI). MI is a therapeutic method that seeks to create a collaborative patient-centered form of communication to strengthen a patient's motivation to change unhealthy behaviors and resistance to treatment. Although originally developed in psychiatry to treat alcohol and substance abuse, the strategy has been used for a variety of conditions, including dietary change, medication adherence, eating disorders, and management of chronic medical disorders. It has also been used in medical settings, including primary care settings. It has never been tested in the Department of Veterans Affairs (VA) health system for CMI, but the concepts of MI can apply to clinicians working with patients who have CMI. They include fostering patient-centered care; creating a sense of collaboration through empathy, support, and shared decision making rather than promoting the clinician's sense of "right"; enhancing rapport by using open-ended questions, well-timed affirmations, and skillful reflective statements; strengthening patient motivation toward behavioral changes that improve health; and avoiding confrontational interactions (Anstiss, 2009; Cole et al., 2011; Lundahl and Burke, 2009; Miller and Rose, 2009).

With regard to effective communication methods for CMI, one qualitative study evaluated the management methods of community-based physicians who were treating patients who had medically unexplained symptoms (Anderson et al., 2008). The strategies considered effective by both physicians and patients included exploring causes and symptoms with tests and referrals, attentive listening, validating complaints, demonstrating commitment to work with the patient over time (including allowing extended office visits and returning telephone calls), providing clear explanations of symptoms and management, and providing explanatory models of the linkage between psychosocial factors and physical symptoms. Strategies that conflicted with proper guidelines and about which physicians had concerns but used nevertheless include ordering potentially unnecessary diagnostic tests, scheduling patients on demand, and prescribing narcotics.

Some strategies for improving the physician–patient relationship have been studied and are of value to all clinicians (Roter and Hall, 1992). First, patient satisfaction is related to the patient's perception of the clinician's humaneness, technical competence, interest in psychosocial factors, and provision of relevant medical information, but too much focus on biomedical issues can have an adverse effect (Bertakis et al., 1991; Hall and Dornan, 1988). Second, some communication methods engage the patient more and ultimately improve clinical outcome, adherence to treatment, reductions in symptoms and pain medication, and shortened hospital stay. These methods include good eye contact, affirmative nods and gestures, a partner-like relationship, closer interpersonal distance, and a gentle tone of voice (Hall et al., 1995; Roter et al., 1987). Finally, clinicians who engage in good communication skills are more apt to like their patients and their work, and their patients are more satisfied (Hall et al., 2002).

Improving the Patient–Clinician Relationship

On the basis of the above observations, the committee offers below several recommendations that it believes will enhance communication and build an effective patient–clinician relationship. Many comments that clinicians use routinely to reassure patients are not helpful for patients who have CMI. For example, "Don't worry, it's nothing serious" or "Your problem is due to stress" will probably have negative consequences for patients who feel that they are not believed or even that they are stigmatized by their disorder (Drossman, 2004); patients may view them as diminishing what they see as real. The clinician needs to accept the reality of the patient's perception as serious and clarify that the symptoms are not due to a psychiatric disorder but rather that the patient has a medical condition that can be psychologically distressing. A comment like "I'd like to order a few tests to be sure there is nothing wrong, but I believe they'll be normal" communicates a mixed message that can be viewed as placating the patient or as indicating that the clinician is practicing defensive medicine (Drossman, 1995). Such comments are not uncommon, because clinicians with a high level of uncertainty are at risk for dealing with CMI by ordering tests more than by making an effort to understand the whole context of the patient's illness (Kappen and van Dulmen, 2008).

An effective patient–clinician relationship occurs through proper interview technique. It is patient-centered, that is, based on creating an environment that encourages the patient to give personal high-quality information, both medical and psychosocial. It occurs through both verbal statements and the behavioral context in which they are made and in relation to facilitative nonverbal behaviors that create a comfortable environment and help to create a partnership of care. The committee recommends several methods and techniques that will enhance the quality of the communication (Chang and Drossman, 2002; Drossman, 1999; Lipkin et al., 1995; Morgan and Engel, 1969; Roter and Hall, 1992).

- *Listen actively.* Clinical data are obtained through an active process of listening, observing, and facilitating. Questions should evolve from what the patient says rather than strictly from a predetermined agenda. If one is uncertain of the patient's response, it helps to restate the information and ask for clarification, and this reaffirms the clinician's commitment to understand.
- *Accept the reality of the disorder.* Many clinicians have difficulty in accepting CMI as a bona fide disorder because there is no biomarker or specific diagnostic test. The difficulty is common in clinicians who work with functional somatic syndromes, such as irritable bowel syndrome, fibromyalgia, and chronic fatigue syndrome. It drives the frequent ordering of tests and the communication of uncertainty. Patients who have CMI desperately want to be believed. The solution is to accept the symptoms as real and to focus on a commitment to work with the patient and his or her illness by listening to understand the patient's illness experience and communicating support.

- *Stay attuned to questioning style and nonverbal messages.* Often, it is not what the clinician says but how he or she says it that makes the difference. Table 6-1 gives examples of several behaviors that either facilitate or inhibit the acquisition of data from the patient. In general, the clinician wants to communicate non-judgmental interest in an environment of comfort, support, and security. Appendix C contains examples of effective and ineffective patient–clinician discussions.

- *Elicit the patient's illness schema.* To negotiate treatment properly, the clinician must identify how the patient understands the illness. In doing so, the clinician can begin a dialogue that will lead to a mutually specified set of goals. For example, even with years of CMI, patients may expect the clinician to diagnose a specific disease and to offer a cure. But the clinician sees it as a chronic disorder that requires continuing management. Those differences must be reconciled if the patient is to accept treatment and cope with the disorder. Several questions can be asked routinely to understand the patient's illness schema:
  — "What brought you here today?"
  — "What do you think you have?"
  — "What worries or concerns do you have?"
  — "What are your thoughts about what I can do to help?"

- *Offer empathy.* The clinician provides empathy by demonstrating an understanding of the patient's pain and distress while maintaining an objective and observant stance. An empathic statement would be, "I can see how difficult it has been for you to manage with all these symptoms" or "I can see how much this has affected your life." Providing empathy improves patient satisfaction and adherence to treatment.

- *Validate the patient's feelings.* When patients disclose personal information, they may experience shame or embarrassment. Therefore, the clinician needs to validate the patient's feelings rather than make personal judgments or close the communication with a quick reassurance or solution (Roter and Hall, 1992). A validating statement to a patient who is feeling stigmatized by others who say that his or her problem is stress-related could be, for example, "I can see you are frustrated when people say that this is due to stress and you know it's real." That type of statement not only validates the patient's feelings but can open the door to further discussion of how the condition can itself be stressful.

- *Be aware of personal thoughts and feelings.* Clinicians can become frustrated when working with patients who have CMI because, unlike better defined medical conditions, CMI lacks a precise diag-

TABLE 6-1 Behaviors That Influence Accurate Data Collection

Behavior	Facilitates	Inhibits
Nonverbal		
Clinical environment	Private, comfortable	Noisy, physical barriers
Eye contact	Frequent	Infrequent or constant
Body posture	Direct, open, relaxed	Body turned, arms folded
Head-nodding	Helpful if well timed	Infrequent, excessive
Body proximity	Close enough to touch	Too close or too distant
Facial expression	Interest, empathy, understanding	Preoccupation, boredom, disapproval
Touching	Helpful when used to communicate empathy	Insincere if not appropriate or properly timed
Verbal		
Question forms	Open-ended to generate hypotheses	Rigid or stereotyped style
	Closed-ended to test hypotheses	Multiple choice or leading questions ("You didn't . . . ?")
	Use of patient's words	Use of unfamiliar words
	Fewer questions and interruptions	More
Question style	Nonjudgmental	Judgmental
	Follows lead of patient's earlier responses	Follows preset agenda or style
	Use of a narrative thread	Unorganized questioning
	Appropriate use of silence	Frequent interruptions
	Appropriate reassurance	Premature or unwarranted reassurance
	Eliciting pertinent psychosocial data in a sensitive and skillful manner	Ignoring psychosocial data or using "probes"

nostic and treatment strategy. Awareness of that limitation can help to minimize reactive or negative behaviors by the clinician. Patients experience physicians' frustration and even rejection. The experience may lead some patients to interact in ways that are perceived as overcautious and "resistant," demanding, or even adversarial. Clinicians may respond defensively or overreact by becoming angry, doing unneeded tests, or overmedicating. Patients' responses can limit the clinician's interest or ability to understand the psychosocial context of the illness. The clinician needs to understand such patient behaviors as responses to deficits in the health care system in providing proper care rather than as patient problems. The clinician must also "tune in" to personal thoughts and feelings (for example, "What is it about this patient's behavior that makes me feel frustrated?") to prevent countertherapeutic responses.

- *Be aware of biases or stereotyping that might lead to unequal treatment.* Bias and stereotyping, although not necessarily conscious, may lead to ethnic disparities and unequal treatment. Such behaviors are more likely to occur in situations where there are clinical uncertainties and time pressures, which often occur when clinicians see patients who have CMI (IOM, 2003).

- *Educate.* Education should be an iterative process. It involves several steps: eliciting the patient's understanding, addressing misunderstandings, providing information that is consistent with the patient's frame of reference or knowledge base, and checking the patient's understanding of what was discussed. Particularly for patients who have CMI, it is important to provide clear explanations of symptoms and treatments in the context of explanatory models that are understandable, are related to treatment, and are consistent with the patient's beliefs. For example, the clinician can explain that because CMI produces many symptoms related to different organ symptoms, the problem (yet to be fully determined) may reside in oversensitivity of nerves or in the brain's failure to "turn down" signals from the nerves. That plausible hypothesis can open the door, for example, to the use of antidepressants as a central analgesic treatment.

- *Reassure.* Patients who have CMI fear serious disease and have negative thoughts and feelings about their condition—helplessness, a lack of control. But reassurance needs to be realistic because a clear understanding of CMI is not yet established. The approach is to identify the patient's worries and concerns, acknowledge or validate them, respond to specific concerns, and avoid "false" reassurances (for example, "Don't worry, everything's fine"), particularly before an initial medical evaluation.

- *Negotiate.* The patient and the clinician must agree on diagnostic and treatment options. The clinician should ask about the patient's experience and about understanding of and interests in various treatments and then provide choices (rather than directives) that are consistent with the patient's beliefs. Negotiation is particularly important in some situations, such as in recommending an anti-depressant (which may be viewed as a "psychiatric" drug rather than a centrally acting analgesic) or in referring the patient to a psychologist for posttraumatic stress disorder or for treatment of other psychologic symptoms.
- *Help the patient to take responsibility.* Patients need to participate actively in their health care, and this can be communicated in several ways. For example, rather than asking the patient, "How are your symptoms today?" one might say, "How are you managing with your symptoms?" The former question tends to leave the clinician with responsibility for dealing with the pain, but the latter acknowledges the patient's role. Another method includes offering any of several treatment approaches and discussing their risks and benefits so that the patient can make the choice.
- *Establish boundaries.* In the care of some patients, "boundaries" regarding frequent telephone calls, unexpected visits, a tendency toward lengthy visits, or unrealistic expectations for care need to be addressed. The task is to present the clinician's needs in a way that is not perceived by the patient as rejecting or belittling. For example, setting limits on time can be accomplished by scheduling brief but regular appointments of fixed duration rather than attempting to extend the time of a particular visit.
- *Provide continuity of care.* Many patients who have CMI feel isolated from the health care system and even from other peers who have medical conditions that are easier to understand. It is valuable to make it clear from the outset that the commitment to care is long-term so that what may be a chronic condition can be managed. Making the commitment to work with the patient avoids patient fears of abandonment.

Additional resources for clinicians to learn more about improving their communication skills are listed in Box 6-1.

BOX 6-1
Additional Resources for Clinicians

Improving communication skills and the patient–clinician interaction is a process that takes more time than is needed for learning content. It also requires self-awareness and feedback from others through training sessions to make such behavioral changes. Clinicians who are interested in acquiring greater skills in this regard should review Web-based video learning programs and attend training courses. Some learning resources are listed below.

DocCom. This is a highly professional self-instruction program that covers basic components of communication and methods to build the patient–clinician relationship and includes numerous models to permit the clinician to address particularly difficult clinical encounters, such as addressing substance abuse, the dying patient, and communication difficulties. This program is one of the best developed and most popular programs designed for teaching medical students, residents, and practitioners. http://webcampus.drexelmed.edu/doccom

American Academy on Communication in Healthcare (AACH). The AACH is one of the oldest organizations composed of an interdisciplinary group of medical educators and clinicians that share a common interest in patient–clinician communication and relationships and in the psychosocial aspects of health care. The AACH provides workshops and courses for clinicians and educators individually or in groups. It maintains an extensive bibliography of articles on patient–clinician communication and a library of educational videos. It focuses on enhancing communication to improve clinical outcomes, lowering risk of malpractice, negotiating and collaborating with patients, mediating challenging patient–clinician encounters, and dealing with uncertainty in diagnosis and treatment. Fellowships are available for advanced training and leadership development. http://www.aachonline.org/

Institute for Healthcare Communication (formerly the Bayer Institute). This organization offers a variety of workshops to help clinicians to develop and hone their communication skills. It also offers books, videos, and practical guides on how to improve communication. Training sessions are available for individuals, in-house consulting for organizations, and "Train the Trainer" programs for advance achievement. http://www.healthcarecomm.org/

NOTE: The resources described here are examples of the types of programs that are available to health care practitioners who are interested in improving their communication skills. They do not constitute an exhaustive list of communication improvement programs.

INFORMATION AND COMMUNICATION TECHNOLOGIES, COMMUNICATION INEQUALITIES, AND CHRONIC MULTISYMPTOM ILLNESS

In addition to patient–clinician encounters, patients' perceptions of illness and of how they are being handled by their clinicians is to a large extent influenced by their interactions with peers, family members, and other important people in their lives. Moreover, patients spend more time outside the encounter and the medical system, and this suggests that there should be other ways to engage patients. Conversations among veterans in social media show veterans' frustration and dissatisfaction with how their illness is being handled but also how conversations outside the medical encounter are probably shaping the perceptions of the veterans (Furey, 2012).

The development of information and communication technologies provides some outstanding opportunities to engage patients and their families more actively in symptom management with a potential for improvement in patient satisfaction and health outcomes. The increasing penetration of Internet use, increasing use of social media, deployment of electronic health records and medical informatics systems, and integration of different digital domains—in short, the emergence of a "cyber-infrastructure"—could, in theory, provide ideal platforms for bringing patients into the loop and encouraging more participatory decision making for those who have CMI (Smits et al., 2008; Viswanath, 2011). Moreover, VA has advanced electronic health records and health informatics architecture that could be exploited to disseminate new models for managing CMI and encouraging patient participation.

Although information and communication technologies provide an important opening for engaging patients, different organizations and groups have different capacity to generate, process, and use information, and different people, such as patients and physicians, have different capacity to access information (Viswanath, 2006). Such communication inequalities have been extensively documented, especially among patients (Cooper and Roter, 2003). For example, patients face major barriers in seeking information outside the medical encounter, and this limits what they learn to information from their physicians (Galarce et al., 2011; Ramanadhan and Viswanath, 2006).

Social class, race, and ethnicity could potentially affect patient–clinician communication, influencing the amount of talk in an encounter, the amount of informative talk, emotional support during the encounter, and question-asking. Possible consequences of this influence are fewer participatory visits, shorter visits, less positive affect, lower satisfaction, lower recall of information, and lower compliance (Cooper and Roter, 2003).

From a patient perspective, the empirical data on access to and use of new information and communication technologies are mixed. National data have repeatedly documented substantial inequalities in accessing and using such technologies as the Internet: Those who have more schooling, higher income, and white-collar occupations enjoy greater access and use than those who have lower incomes, less schooling, and manual occupations (Blake et al., 2011; Kontos et al., 2010; Viswanath, 2011; Viswanath and Ackerson, 2011). VA's deployment of patient portals and health records and its relatively advanced deployment of health information technology warrant an examination of how veterans use the Internet. There are few data on the issue. One national study that oversampled veterans showed that only half of veterans used the Internet and that about 29% of all veterans who responded to the survey used it for health (McInnes et al., 2010). In contrast, national data showed that 61% of those who access the Internet have accessed health information (Fox and Jones, 2009).

Although the "digital divide" is real and persistent, developments in information and communication technologies and new consumer informatics platforms offer considerable opportunity to reach out to veterans and engage them and to build a collaborative platform between VA and veterans. A key platform is social media. Social media are a product of the larger Web 2.0 developments that, unlike the prior version of the Web, engage users more actively and encourage interactivity. Social media facilitate participation through user-generated content, an approach that is more participatory. Social media platforms are varied and include those which encourage collaboration, such as Wikipedia; blogs and microblogs, such as Twitter; social networking, such as Facebook; content communities, such as YouTube; games; and virtual social worlds. The penetration of social media has been fast and furious, and they have overtaken the growth of other platforms on the Web. Almost 66% of online adults use social media platforms, according to the Pew Internet & American Life Project, and much of the use is focused on staying in touch with friends and family members (Pew Research Center, 2012).

More germane to the present discussion is the fact that, unlike the digital divide that is characterized by lower online access and use by those in a lower socioeconomic groups, social networking use is not patterned by class, race, or ethnicity (see Table 6-2). In fact, minority groups are more likely to use social media, and income and schooling matter much less (Kontos et al., 2010; Pew Research Center, 2012). Age is one important determinant: older groups, particularly those over 65 years old, are much less likely than younger groups to use social media.

In short, the participatory and engaging nature of social media provides one optimal platform for VA to use to reach and engage veterans who have CMI. Many veterans are already active on social media (Furey, 2012).

TABLE 6-2 Characteristics of Users of Social Media

Characteristic	Fraction of Internet Users,[a] %
Sex	
Men	63
Women	75*
Age, years	
18–29	92***
30–49	73**
50–64	57*
65+	38
Race and Ethnicity	
White, non-Hispanic	68
Black, non-Hispanic	68
Hispanic (English- and Spanish-speaking)	72
Household Income	
Less than $30,000	73*
$30,000–49,000	66
$50,000–74,000	66
$75,000+	74**
Education Level	
Less than high school	65
High school graduate	65
Some college	73*
College+	72*

NOTES: Table shows percentage of Internet users in each group who use social-networking sites. An asterisk indicates statistically significant differences between rows. Extra asterisks mean differences with all rows with lower figures within each category.
[a]Internet users make up 66% of US population.
SOURCE: Reproduced with permission from Pew Research Center's Internet & American Life Project.

However, the grassroots and participatory approach of social media warrants a shift away from the "command and control" approach that institutions have traditionally taken. To achieve that shift, VA should develop more active social media strategies to work with veterans who have CMI.

There are opportunities for VA to disseminate new guidelines and to change clinician behaviors as well as engage patients. There are no simple or precise models of dissemination, but the lessons from earlier experiences of dissemination and implementation offer some useful pointers. Diffusion (a passive process that involves unplanned spread of evidence-based information with little attention to specificity in defining the target audience or to customization of the information itself) and dissemination (a purposive flow of customized information toward a well-defined target audience) of guidelines and innovations make clinicians aware of them and prepared to adopt them. Diffusion and dissemination by themselves are unlikely to lead to behavior change. Behavior change requires more active implementation strategies that focus at three levels. At the system level, there is a need for the development and deployment of decision-support systems that are user-friendly and customized to local needs and that find support in local organizations. A greater flexibility in modifying systems and procedures to support adoption of new CMI guidelines, support from management, and constant monitoring and evaluation in the form of continuous quality improvement are key determinants in the adoption of new guidelines to treat for CMI. Active communication and marketing will help to facilitate organizational changes and to ease barriers. A continuous quality-improvement approach will also ensure constant feedback to inform the implementation of and changes in CMI treatment guidelines.

As discussed in more depth in Chapter 7, at the clinician and network level, local champions and peer networks offer a supportive setting for learning skills informally, provide role models, and create the right environment for adopting new guidelines. Investment in the training of and incentives for clinicians and care teams will facilitate adoption and ease barriers.

In addition to "push" factors that actively disseminate education and information, working with patients will ensure that "pull" factors that involve patient engagement impel the adoption. Patient engagement can be engendered by taking advantage of social media platforms and combining consumer informatics technologies with VA's fast-developing health-informatics platforms.

Finally, it is important to remind ourselves that communication inequalities could potentially deter patients from taking full advantage of new information and communication technologies, so efforts should be made to ensure that veterans who do not access the Internet can be reached in other ways.

REFERENCES

Aiarzaguena, J. M., G. Grandes, I. Gaminde, A. Salazar, A. Sanchez, and J. Arino. 2007. A randomized controlled clinical trial of a psychosocial and communication intervention carried out by GPS for patients with medically unexplained symptoms. *Psychological Medicine* 37(2):283-294.

Aiarzaguena, J. M., I. Gaminde, G. Grandes, A. Salazar, I. Alonso, and A. Sanchez. 2009. Somatisation in primary care: Experiences of primary care physicians involved in a training program and in a randomised controlled trial. *BMC Family Practice* 10:73.

Anderson, M., A. Hartz, T. Nordin, M. Rosenbaum, R. Noyes, P. James, J. Ely, N. Agarwal, and S. Anderson. 2008. Community physicians' strategies for patients with medically unexplained symptoms. *Family Medicine* 40(2):111-118.

Anstiss, T. 2009. Motivational interviewing in primary care. *Journal of Clinical Psychology in Medical Settings* 16(1):87-93.

Bertakis, K. D., D. Roter, and S. M. Putnam. 1991. The relationship of physician medical interview style to patient satisfaction. *Journal of Family Practice* 32(2):175-181.

Blake, K., S. Flynt-Wallington, and K. Viswanath. 2011. Health communication channel preferences by class, race, and place. In *Health Communication: Building the Evidence Base in Cancer Control*, edited by G. Kreps. Cresskill, NJ: Hampton Press. Pp. 149-174.

Chang, L., and D. A. Drossman. 2002. Optimizing patient care: The psychosocial interview in the irritable bowel syndrome. *Clinical Perspectives in Gastroenterology* 5(6):336-341.

Christianson, J. B., L. H. Warrick, M. Finch, and W. B. Jonas. 2012. *Physician Communication with Patients: Research Findings and Challenges*. Ann Arbor: The University of Michigan Press.

Cole, S. V., M. Bogenschutz, and D. Hungerford. 2011. Motivational interviewing and psychiatry: Use in addiction treatment, risky drinking and routine practice. *FOCUS* 9:42-54.

Cooper, L., and D. Roter. 2003. Patient–provider communication: The effect of race and ethnicity on process and outcomes of healthcare. In *Unequal Treatment: Confronting Racial and Ethnic Disparities in Health Care*, edited by B. Smedley, A. Stith and A. Nelson. Washington, DC: The National Academies Press. Pp. 552-593.

Drossman, D. A. 1995. Diagnosing and treating patients with refractory functional gastrointestinal disorders. *Annals of Internal Medicine* 123(9):688-697.

Drossman, D. A. 1999. The physician-patient relationship. In *Approach to the Patient with Chronic Gastrointestinal Disorders*, edited by E. Corazziari. Milan: Messaggi. Pp. 133-139.

Drossman, D. A. 2004. Functional abdominal pain syndrome. *Clinical Gastroenterology & Hepatology* 2(5):353-365.

Epstein, R. M., C. G. Shields, S. C. Meldrum, K. Fiscella, J. Carroll, P. A. Carney, and P. R. Duberstein. 2006. Physicians' responses to patients' medically unexplained symptoms. *Psychosomatic Medicine* 68(2):269-276.

Fazekas, C., F. Matzer, E. R. Greimel, G. Moser, M. Stelzig, W. Langewitz, B. Loewe, W. Pieringer, and E. Jandl-Jager. 2009. Psychosomatic medicine in primary care: Influence of training. *Wiener Klinische Wochenschrift* 121(13-14):446-453.

Fortin, A. H., VI, F. C. Dwamena, R. M. Frankel, and R. C. Smith. 2012. *Smith's Patient-Centered Interviewing: An Evidence-Based Method*. 3rd ed. New York: The McGraw-Hill Companies, Inc.

Fox, S., and S. Jones. 2009. *The Social Life of Health Information*. Pew Charitable Trusts. http://www.pewinternet.org/Reports/2011/Social-Life-of-Health-Info.aspx

Friedberg, F., S. J. Sohl, and P. J. Halperin. 2008. Teaching medical students about medically unexplained illnesses: A preliminary study. *Medical Teacher* 30(6):618-621.

Frostholm, L., P. Fink, E. Oernboel, K. S. Christensen, T. Toft, F. Olesen, and J. Weinman. 2005. The uncertain consultation and patient satisfaction: The impact of patients' illness perceptions and a randomized controlled trial on the training of physicians' communication skills. *Psychosomatic Medicine* 67(6):897-905.

Furey, P. 2012 (unpublished). *Analysis of the Social Media Discussion of Chronic Multisymptom Illness in Veterans of the Iraq and Afghanistan Wars*. Analysis commissioned by the Committee on Gulf War and Health: Treatment of Chronic Multisymptom Illness, Institute of Medicine, Washington, DC.

Galarce, E. M., S. Ramanadhan, J. Weeks, E. C. Schneider, S. W. Gray, and K. Viswanath. 2011. Class, race, ethnicity and information needs in post-treatment cancer patients. *Patient Education and Counseling* 85(3):432-439.

Hall, J. A., and M. C. Dornan. 1988. What patients like about their medical care and how often they are asked: A meta-analysis of the satisfaction literature. *Social Science & Medicine* 27(9):935-939.

Hall, J. A., J. A. Harrigan, and R. Rosenthal. 1995. Nonverbal behavior in clinician patient interaction. *Applied & Preventive Psychology* 4(1):21-37.

Hall, J. A., T. G. Horgan, T. S. Stein, and D. L. Roter. 2002. Liking in the physician-patient relationship. *Patient Education and Counseling* 48(1):69-77.

Hunt, S. C., R. D. Richardson, C. C. Engel, D. C. Atkins, and M. McFall. 2004. Gulf War veterans' illnesses: A pilot study of the relationship of illness beliefs to symptom severity and functional health status. *Journal of Occupational and Environmental Medicine* 46(8):818-827.

IOM (Institute of Medicine). 2003. *Unequal Treatment: Confronting Racial and Ethnic Disparities in Health Care.* Washington, DC: The National Academies Press.

Kappen, T., and S. van Dulmen. 2008. General practitioners' responses to the initial presentation of medically unexplained symptoms: A quantitative analysis. *BioPsychoSocial Medicine* 2:22.

Kontos, E. Z., K. Viswanath, K. M. Emmons, and E. Puleo. 2010. Communications inequalities and public health implications of adult social networking site use in the United States. *Journal of Health Communication* 15(3):216-235.

Larisch, A., A. Schweickhardt, M. Wirsching, and K. Fritzsche. 2004. Psychosocial interventions for somatizing patients by the general practitioner: A randomized controlled trial. *Journal of Psychosomatic Research* 57(6):507-514.

Levinson, W., D. L. Roter, J. P. Mullooly, V. T. Dull, and R. M. Frankel. 1997. Physician-patient communication: The relationship with malpractice claims among primary care physicians and surgeons. *Journal of the American Medical Association* 277(7):553-559.

Lipkin, M., S. M. Putnam, and A. Laare. 1995. *The Medical Interview: Clinical Care, Education, and Research.* 1st ed. New York: Springer-Verlag.

Lundahl, B., and B. L. Burke. 2009. The effectiveness and applicability of motivational interviewing: A practice-friendly review of four meta-analyses. *Journal of Clinical Psychology* 65(11):1232-1245.

Makoul, G. 2001. Essential elements of communication in medical encounters: The Kalamazoo Consensus Statement. *Academic Medicine Journal of the Association of American Medical Colleges* 76(4):390-393.

Margalit, A. P. A., and A. El-Ad. 2008. Costly patients with unexplained medical symptoms: A high-risk population. *Patient Education & Counseling* 70(2):173-178.

McInnes, D. K., A. L. Gifford, L. E. Kazis, and T. H. Wagner. 2010. Disparities in health-related Internet use by US veterans: Results from a national survey. *Informatics in Primary Care* 18(1):59-68.

Miller, W. R., and G. S. Rose. 2009. Toward a theory of motivational interviewing. *American Psychologist* 64(6):527-537.

Morgan, W. L., and G. L. Engel. 1969. The approach to the medical interview. In *The Clinical Approach to the Patient*, edited by W. L. Morgan and G. L. Engel. Philadelphia: W. B. Saunders. Pp. 26-79.

Morriss, R., C. Dowrick, P. Salmon, S. Peters, G. Dunn, A. Rogers, B. Lewis, H. Charles-Jones, J. Hogg, R. Clifford, C. Rigby, and L. Gask. 2007. Cluster randomised controlled trial of training practices in reattribution for medically unexplained symptoms. *British Journal of Psychiatry* 191:536-542.

Nettleton, S., I. Watt, L. O'Malley, and P. Duffey. 2005. Understanding the narratives of people who live with medically unexplained illness. *Patient Education & Counseling* 56(2):205-210.

olde Hartman, T. C., M. S. Borghuis, P. L. B. J. Lucassen, F. A. van de Laar, A. E. Speckens, and C. van Weel. 2009. Medically unexplained symptoms, somatisation disorder and hypochondriasis: Course and prognosis. A systematic review. *Journal of Psychosomatic Research* 66(5):363-377.

Ostbye, T., K. S. H. Yarnall, K. M. Krause, K. I. Pollak, M. Gradison, and J. L. Michener. 2005. Is there time for management of patients with chronic diseases in primary care? *Annals of Family Medicine* 3(3):209-214.

Pew Research Center. 2012. *Pew Internet & American Life Project.* http://pewinternet.org/ (accessed November 29, 2012).

Pols, R. G., and M. W. Battersby. 2008. Coordinated care in the management of patients with unexplained physical symptoms: Depression is a key issue. *Medical Journal of Australia* 188(12 Suppl):S133-S137.

Ramanadhan, S., and K. Viswanath. 2006. Health and the information nonseeker: A profile. *Health Communication* 20(2):131-139.

Rasmussen, N. H., J. W. Furst, D. M. Swenson-Dravis, D. C. Agerter, A. J. Smith, M. A. Baird, and S. S. Cha. 2006. Innovative reflecting interview: Effect on high-utilizing patients with medically unexplained symptoms. *Disease Management* 9(6):349-359.

Ring, A., C. Dowrick, G. Humphris, and P. Salmon. 2004. Do patients with unexplained physical symptoms pressurise general practitioners for somatic treatment? A qualitative study. *British Medical Journal* 328(7447):1057.

Rosendal, M., F. Olesen, P. Fink, T. Toft, I. Sokolowski, and F. Bro. 2007. A randomized controlled trial of brief training in the assessment and treatment of somatization in primary care: Effects on patient outcome. *General Hospital Psychiatry* 29(4):364-373.

Roter, D. L., and J. A. Hall. 1989. Physicians interviewing styles and medical information obtained from patients. *Journal of General Internal Medicine* 2(5):325-329.

Roter, D. L., and J. A. Hall. 1992. *Doctors Talking with Patients/Patients Talking with Doctors: Improving Communication in Medical Visits.* 1st ed. Westport, CT: Greenwood Publishing Group.

Roter, D. L., J. A. Hall, and N. R. Katz. 1987. Relations between physicians' behaviors and analogue patients' satisfaction, recall, and impressions. *Medical Care* 25(5):437-451.

Roter, D. L., J. A. Hall, D. E. Kern, L. R. Barker, K. A. Cole, and R. P. Roca. 1995. Improving physicians' interviewing skills and reducing patients' emotional distress: A randomized clinical trial. *Archives of Internal Medicine* 155(17):1877-1884.

Salmon, P., G. M. Humphris, A. Ring, J. C. Davies, and C. F. Dowrick. 2007. Primary care consultations about medically unexplained symptoms: Patient presentations and doctor responses that influence the probability of somatic intervention. *Psychosomatic Medicine* 69(6):571-577.

Schilte, A. F., P. J. Portegijs, A. H. Blankenstein, H. E. van Der Horst, M. B. Latour, J. T. van Eijk, and J. A. Knottnerus. 2001. Randomised controlled trial of disclosure of emotionally important events in somatisation in primary care. *British Medical Journal* 323(7304):86.

Smith, R. C., and F. C. Dwamena. 2007. Classification and diagnosis of patients with medically unexplained symptoms. *Journal of General Internal Medicine* 22(5):685-691.

Smith, R. C., C. Lein, C. Collins, J. S. Lyles, B. Given, F. C. Dwamena, J. Coffey, A. Hodges, J. C. Gardiner, J. Goddeeris, and C. Given. 2003. Treating patients with medically unexplained symptoms in primary care. *Journal of General Internal Medicine* 18(6):478-489.

Smith, R. C., J. S. Lyles, J. C. Gardiner, C. Sirbu, A. Hodges, C. Collins, F. C. Dwamena, C. Lein, C. Given, B. Given, and J. Goddeeris. 2006. Primary care clinicians treat patients with medically unexplained symptoms: A randomized controlled trial. *Journal of General Internal Medicine* 21(7):671-677.

Smith, R. C., J. C. Gardiner, Z. Luo, S. Schooley, L. Lamerato, and K. Rost. 2009. Primary care physicians treat somatization. *Journal of General Internal Medicine* 24(7):829-832.

Smits, F. T. M., K. A. Wittkampf, A. H. Schene, P. J. E. Bindels, and H. C. P. M. Van Weert. 2008. Interventions on frequent attenders in primary care. A systematic literature review. *Scandinavian Journal of Primary Health Care* 26(2):111-116.

Toft, T., M. Rosendal, E. Ornbol, F. Olesen, L. Frostholm, and P. Fink. 2010. Training general practitioners in the treatment of functional somatic symptoms: Effects on patient health in a cluster-randomised controlled trial (the Functional Illness in Primary Care study). *Psychotherapy & Psychosomatics* 79(4):227-237.

Van Der Feltz-Cornelis, C., P. Van Oppen, H. Ader, and R. Van Dyck. 2006. Collaborative care for medically unexplained physical symptoms in general practice. *Huisarts en Wetenschap* 49(7):342-347.

Viswanath, K. 2006. Public communications and its role in reducing and eliminating health disparities. In *Examining the Health Disparities Research Plan of the National Institutes of Health: Unfinished Business*, edited by G. E. Thomson, F. Mitchell, and M. B. Williams. Washington, DC: Institute of Medicine. Pp. 215-253.

Viswanath, K. 2011. Cyberinfrastructure: An extraordinary opportunity to bridge health and communication inequalities? *American Journal of Preventive Medicine* 40(5S2):S245-S248.

Viswanath, K., and L. K. Ackerson. 2011. Race, ethnicity, language, social class, and health communication inequalities: A nationally-representative cross-sectional study. *PloS One* 6(1).

7

Implementation and Models of Care for Veterans Who Have Chronic Multisymptom Illness

As previously described, nearly all veterans who have chronic multisymptom illness (CMI) have comorbid illnesses—illnesses that are themselves multisymptomatic and that overlap with CMI in complex and highly variable ways. The most common chronic condition in the United States, and probably the world, is multimorbidity (Tinetti et al., 2012), and this is especially true for patients who have CMI. Even though there may be evidence-based treatments for one or more of these conditions, the committee believes that a treatment plan consisting simply of the sum of these practice guidelines will be altogether inadequate and is ill-advised. An integrated approach to care is required. There is a fundamental difference between managing a disease or a condition and caring for a person who has one or more conditions—just as there is a fundamental difference between a clinical practice guideline (CPG) and a personal care plan. Anecdotal evidence suggests that simply adhering to multiple CPGs often is not effective for managing chronic conditions with multiple morbidities such as CMI and can result in incomplete care and decrease patient satisfaction, and increase the likelihood of overtreatment and adverse side effects. Each personal care plan will be peculiar to the individual veteran (although crafted from the therapeutic elements outlined in Chapters 4 and 5), will change, and will almost always be complex and detailed. A clinician caring for a veteran who has CMI faces a daunting and time-consuming task that cannot always be accomplished in the course of an ordinary primary care visit and can hardly be implemented by a single clinician; it generally takes a team approach and specific expertise. Special consideration must be given to the resources and the organization—the system of care—that are marshaled for the management of CMI patients.

This chapter presents a patient-centered management approach for veterans who have CMI. It begins by describing some of the current capabilities of the Department of Veterans Affairs (VA) for managing the health of veterans. It identifies inadequacies of existing VA models of care for veterans who have CMI and recommends a general approach to the management of such veterans. The chapter next describes models of care used by other organizations to manage CMI patients. Building on information presented in Chapter 6, it ends with a discussion of how information about managing CMI might be disseminated to VA clinicians and patients.

MODELS OF CARE FOR CHRONIC MULTISYMPTOM ILLNESS IN THE DEPARTMENT OF VETERANS AFFAIRS HEALTH CARE SYSTEM

Veterans use the full array of health care benefits and systems for their care: the Veterans Health Administration (VHA); TRICARE, the Department of Defense (DOD) health care program for active-duty, reserve, and retired armed forces personnel; Medicare; and private care. Fewer than 20% of all veterans receive their health care exclusively in VHA facilities, about one-third of veterans use Medicare benefits, and almost half use both (Hynes et al., 2007; Petersen et al., 2010; Stroupe et al., 2005; West et al., 2008). The distribution among the health care system of veterans who have CMI is not known, nor is there any difference in the pathway of care between veterans of the 1991 Gulf War and veterans of the Iraq and Afghanistan wars (Operation Iraqi Freedom, Operation New Dawn, and Operation Enduring Freedom).

More than 8 million veterans are enrolled in VHA (Walters, 2011). In FY 2009, the number of pre–September 2001 Gulf War–era veterans receiving health care through VHA was 571,656 (VA, 2011d).[1] That number represents 8.7% of the total Gulf War–era veteran cohort. Of the pre–September 2001 Gulf War–era veterans receiving care from VHA, 145,832 were deployed to the Persian Gulf and 110,487 of the deployed personnel were active participants in the Gulf War. Inpatient care in VHA facilities was used by 24,578 pre–September 2001 Gulf War–era veterans in FY 2009, and outpatient care was used by 540,802 Gulf War–era veterans in the same year. About 55% of veterans of the Iraq and Afghanistan wars (834,463 veterans) have used VHA health care services since October 2001

---

[1]For this case, Gulf War–era veterans are defined as military personnel who served on active duty during August 2, 1990–September 10, 2001. Not all Gulf War–era veterans were deployed to the Persian Gulf or were Gulf War participants.

(VA, 2012a). Among those Iraq and Afghanistan war veterans who have sought care at VHA facilities, about 94% have used only outpatient services and about 6% have been hospitalized at least once (VA, 2012a).

VHA has substantial experience in treating patients who have chronic illnesses. Its patients have a higher prevalence of the eight most common chronic health conditions than do patients who are using TRICARE and private plans (Gibson et al., 2009), not including CMI. As indicated above, information is not available on the number of veterans who have CMI and receive their care from VHA or elsewhere.

Postdeployment Patient-Aligned Care Team Program

Gulf War veterans have begun to enter the VHA system by being assigned to a postdeployment patient-aligned care team (PD-PACT) (Hunt, 2012). A PD-PACT serves as a veteran's medical home in VHA. The move to a medical-home model is relatively recent in VHA and implementation is ongoing (Reisinger et al., 2012). VHA's implementation of this model of care compares favorably with implementation in most civilian practices and systems, in which the transition to patient-centered medical homes is still in the early stages of implementation. VHA has established principles and guidelines for the implementation of PACTs, educated its clinicians about the principles, and assigned champions to lead the implementation effort (VA, 2012j). It is important to note that this pathway to care did not exist when military personnel were returning from the 1991 Gulf War and entering the VHA system. The 1991 Gulf War veterans are now being served by PD-PACTs, but their enrollment rates have been highly variable among settings (VA, 2012e). The plan is for assignment to a PD-PACT to begin after a postdeployment comprehensive health examination and a postdeployment disability determination. At some sites, the wait time for the two steps is extremely long, sometimes more than a year. That is frustrating for veterans, who sometimes seek care elsewhere; it also compromises PACT primary care clinicians' ability to render high-quality care.

Each PD-PACT is overseen by a project manager. Other team members can include primary care clinicians, nursing-care managers, mental health clinicians, social workers, and others who have expertise in such subjects as brain injury and physical rehabilitation. The number, specialty types, relative availability, and extent of integration into the primary care team of specialty-team members vary widely from clinic to clinic; VHA currently assigns behavioral-health clinicians to PACTs in VA medical centers (VAMCs) and outpatient clinics that have more than 5,000 primary care patients, and many smaller clinics also have behavioral clinicians on PACT teams. A veteran being cared for is considered a member of the team. The goal of the PD-PACT model is to provide comprehensive, integrated care, including follow-up health care, education, and training (Reisinger et al., 2012). Postdeployment integrated care services are in place in 79% of VAMCs and 35% of community-based outpatient clinics (Hunt, 2012), but the extent to which these teams actually function as teams and contain all the necessary expertise is highly variable. Under ideal circumstances, PD-PACT members work together as a coherent team, but many PD-PACT members operate as consultants without a continuing commitment to patients' care plans and without close communication with other PACT members. Some 84% of VAMCs have clinical experts who can provide clinical guidance for veterans in the context of their continuing primary care (Hunt, 2012).

Educational Materials

VHA provides extensive educational materials to patients and their families about such topics as environmental exposures, associated adverse health outcomes, and techniques for self-management of symptoms. For example, materials are available on controlled-breathing techniques (VA, 2009a), complementary and integrative medicine (VA, 2011b), using exercise to manage chronic pain and fatigue (VA, 2011c), and medically unexplained symptoms (VA, 2011e). Materials also are produced for clinicians (for example, a resource guide on helping patients self-manage their symptoms) (VA, 2009c).

Clinical Practice Guidelines

VHA has a CPG for the management of veterans who have symptoms that remain unexplained after appropriate medical assessment (VA and DOD, 2001b).[2] In addition, VHA has developed CPGs for a number of relevant conditions, including postdeployment health and common comorbidities and conditions that have overlapping symptoms, such as major depressive disorder, posttraumatic stress disorder, traumatic brain injury, and chronic pain (Chou et al., 2007; VA and DOD, 2001a, 2009a,b,c, 2010a,b). The CPG on medically unexplained symptoms provides a general approach for managing CMI patients. For example, the key points made in the CPG (VA and DOD, 2001b) are to

- Obtain a thorough medical history, physical examination, and medical record review.

---

[2]VA has plans to update its 2001 CPG on medically unexplained symptoms (personal communication, C. Cassidy, Office of Quality and Safety, Department of Veterans Affairs, March 19, 2012).

- Minimize low-yield diagnostic testing.
- Identify treatable causes (conditions) for the patient's symptoms.
- Determine if the patient can be classified as having chronic multi-symptom illness (CMI) (that is, has two or more symptom clusters: pain, fatigue, cognitive dysfunction, or sleep disturbance).
- Negotiate treatment options and establish collaboration with the patient.
- Provide appropriate patient and family education.
- Maximize the use of nonpharmacologic therapies:
  — Graded aerobic exercise with close monitoring.
  — Cognitive behavioral therapy.
- Empower patients to take an active role in their recovery.

The guidelines are useful and appropriate, and VHA has published its method for disseminating and implementing its CPGs in VHA clinics (Nicholas et al., 2001; VA and DOD, 2011).

VHA has also published a study guide (not a full CPG) for clinicians on caring for veterans of the 1991 Gulf War (VA, 2011a). It includes information on exposures of concern to veterans of the 1991 Gulf War and instructions for conducting an exposure assessment of veterans. It also contains a section on undiagnosed and unexplained illnesses, including information about CMI.

Specialty Care Access Network

Although VHA has 153 medical centers and more than 900 outpatient clinics nationwide, not all veterans have easy access to VHA facilities (Reisinger et al., 2012). Accordingly, VHA developed a specialty care access network (SCAN) to bring specialty care to veterans who live in rural and other underserved areas, generally areas that do not have VAMCs (VA, 2012e). SCAN is modeled after Project ECHO (Extension for Community Healthcare Outcomes), a program developed by the University of New Mexico Health System. The mission of Project ECHO is to develop the capacity to treat chronic, common, and complex diseases in rural and underserved areas safely and effectively and to monitor outcomes (Arora et al., 2011). The program works by bringing ECHO network specialists with the medical expertise necessary for the condition being addressed into otherwise isolated primary care practices. After an initial in-person orientation, a team meets weekly via video conference to present and discuss patients and to formulate care plans. The program fits well into the medical home model by augmenting comprehensiveness, improving continuity and coordination of care, and enhancing quality and safety of care. An important element of the ECHO program is teaching and implementing concepts of team management of patients (Katzman, 2012).

VHA adopted the SCAN-ECHO program in 2010 and contracted with Project ECHO to leverage technology and use case-based learning to educate its primary care physicians in chronic pain management and other specialty care topics. Eleven regional VAMCs are using the SCAN-ECHO program. In addition, VAMCs in Denver, Colorado; Richmond, Virginia; Cleveland, Ohio; Albuquerque, New Mexico; greater Los Angeles, California; Salem, Massachusetts; Portland, Oregon; and New Haven, Connecticut, are now replicating the Project ECHO chronic pain program, and clinicians in their regions are calling in each week for consultations related to pain management (VA, 2012e).

War-Related Illness and Injury Study Centers

Under a congressional mandate, VA established war-related illness and injury study centers (WRIISCs) in 2001 to serve combat veterans who had unexplained illnesses (Lincoln et al., 2006). Three WRIISCs are operating in East Orange, New Jersey; Palo Alto, California; and Washington, DC. The WRIISCs are multidisciplinary centers of excellence to which veterans who are severely afflicted with CMI can be referred. They also are charged with conducting research on CMI and its constituent symptoms and with creating and disseminating educational materials for veterans, their families, and clinicians (Lincoln et al., 2006; VA, 2012l).

Veterans may be referred to a WRIISC by their clinicians. Referrals generally come about because a veteran has a complex medical history of no known etiology, treatments have resulted in little or no symptom improvement, deployment-related environmental exposures may have occurred, or the veteran is not improving and further local expertise is unavailable (Reinhard, 2012). Veterans in a WRIISC are evaluated by a multidisciplinary team that conducts a comprehensive health assessment and formulates a comprehensive personal care plan aimed at managing symptoms and improving functional health; the plan is implemented in the WRIISC and given to the referring clinicians (Lincoln et al., 2006). As of 2012, the WRIISCs' clinical programs have conducted health assessments of about 1,000 veterans (Reinhard, 2012).

Patient-Centered Medical Care and the Office of Cultural Transformation

VHA has established an office of Patient Centered Care and Cultural Transformation (Petzel, 2012; VA, 2012g,h). The goal of the office is to develop personal, patient-centered models of care for veterans who receive their health care at VHA facilities. There will be greater focus on providing team-based care and integrative approaches throughout VHA. The office seeks to address the "full range of physical, emotional, mental, social, spiritual, and environmental influences" on veterans (VA, 2012g).

Summary of Models of Care in the
Department of Veterans Affairs Health Care System

VHA has developed extensive infrastructure and support for veterans who have CMI and the clinicians who care for them: multispecialty teams, practice guidelines, training and educational materials for clinicians and patients, access to consultants when they are not available locally, support for such elements of implementation as practice champions, the basic structure of a system of stepped care, and more. The infrastructure is remarkable and far outstrips the corresponding elements of the civilian health care system, which is generally much less developed. All those efforts notwithstanding, however, veterans who have CMI will remain seriously underserved, and their clinicians will remain unable to serve them adequately, until additional measures are put into place. Clinical guidelines for chronic conditions are extraordinarily difficult to implement, and their implementation follows a set of rules and principles that are just now becoming understood. CPGs assume a degree of uniformity of presentation and severity and the availability of time, training, and personnel that are not always available even in the most dedicated and highest-quality settings. But the patients present with highly variable and ever-changing symptom constellations—with a spectrum of severity ranging from just barely symptomatic to profoundly disabled—in a highly variable and constantly changing clinical environment. Thus, the treatment burden of and need for care coordination is not uniform among clinical settings. Finally, and most important, even in settings where it is possible to bring a high degree of standardization, the team members themselves—their seniority, previous experiences, personalities, team "chemistry," and response to the particular local leaders—constitute a source of irreducible variation that must be taken into account in the implementation process. Local practice coaches and other local resources are almost always necessary for successful implementation. The issue of implementation will be addressed after a description of the veterans' experience of care.

GULF WAR VETERANS' EXPERIENCE OF CARE

Patient Satisfaction

Despite the extensive efforts devoted to improving care for veterans who have CMI, some Gulf War veterans have expressed frustration and anger about what they consider to be subpar care from VHA (public comments to the committee, December 17, 2011, and February 1, 2012; Furey, 2012). Often, they do not believe that VHA clinicians take their symptoms seriously, and they get the impression that the clinicians believe that their health problems are mental in origin.

Gulf War veterans report less satisfaction with waiting-room time, copayment or costs, courtesy of office staff, and clinician time than World War II veterans (Harada et al., 2002). Differences in several other variables were not significant—number of days waited for an appointment, how easy it is to get around a facility, clinician skill, and overall satisfaction. Harada et al. (2002) found that veterans who used both VHA and non-VHA facilities ("dual users") were less satisfied overall with their outpatient care than were veterans who used only VHA or only non-VHA facilities.

In a study that compared veterans' satisfaction with types of clinicians in VHA facilities, satisfaction scores increased as the numbers of nurse practitioners increased (Budzi et al., 2010). Veterans are more satisfied with nurse-practitioners who were trained in particular skills, such as paying attention to and providing for the patient's educational needs, individualized care, and active listening.

Health status is significantly associated with patient satisfaction in veterans who use VHA outpatient care (Ren et al., 2001). Mental health status correlates more strongly with patient satisfaction than does physical health status. In general, veterans who are healthier are more likely to be satisfied with their care. Satisfaction can be both a consequence and a determinant of health status; in the study by Ren et al. (2001), health status seemed to be more of a determinant of patient satisfaction than the reverse.

Veterans who had chronic illnesses and experienced greater satisfaction with VHA were less likely to seek care elsewhere after discharge from active duty (Stroupe et al., 2005). Greater dissatisfaction at baseline led to a greater probability that veterans would later go outside the VHA system, thereby seeding the civilian primary care sector with unhappy veterans who had CMI. Veterans older than 65 years old are more likely to use non-VHA health care facilities than younger veterans; this may be due to the older veterans' Medicare eligibility.

Female veterans reported scores similar to those of male veterans on most dimensions of outpatient satisfaction with VHA facilities after adjustment for a number of demographic attributes (Wright et al., 2006).

Access to Care

On discharge from the active-duty military, a portion of veterans (8.57 million of a total of about 22.23 million in FY 2011) enroll in the VA health care system (VA, 2012d). To balance demand with resources, VHA uses health care enrollment priority groups (see Box 7-1). The threshold for enrollment changes on the basis of available resources.

The amount of time it takes veterans to get an appointment to visit a VHA clinician varies widely from one clinic to another. Harada et al. (2002) reported that one of veterans' highest points of dissatisfaction with VHA was the wait time for an appointment. In 2010, nearly all primary care appointments at VHA facilities occurred within 30 days of the desired date (Walters, 2011). In 2011, the standard for primary care appointments was changed to 14 days, which was already the standard for mental health appointments. Data were not available to describe whether VHA has been able to meet the 14-day standard. However, a review by the VA Office of the Inspector General (VA-OIG) found that many veterans waited more than 14 days *past* their desired appointment date for their mental health appointments (VA, 2012k). In addition, the VA-OIG determined that the "VHA overstated its success in providing veterans new and follow-up appointments for treatment within 14 days." The principal reasons for wait times to exceed the established standard were inconsistent application of procedures by VHA schedulers and too few mental health clinicians on staff.

Location of VHA facilities affects veterans' access to care. VHA has over 1,000 facilities, including VAMCs and outpatient clinics, but they are geographically dispersed, and not every veteran has easy access to one (Reisinger et al., 2012). For example, 43% of veterans live in rural areas that may not be readily served by VHA facilities (Walters, 2011). A VA review on interventions to improve access to care found that as distance from a VHA facility increased there was decreased use of outpatient services and that the greatest decrease occurred for distances up to 60 miles from the facility (Kehle et al., 2011). The relationship between facility distance from home and care use was consistent for physical health and mental health appointments. VHA is developing strategies to bring health care to rural veterans through such means as mobile health clinics, telehealth programs, and health care partnerships (Walters, 2011).

In its review, VA evaluated whether integration of primary care and mental health care would increase veterans' access to mental health services (Kehle et al., 2011). Both integrating mental health services into primary care clinics and offering primary care in mental health clinics showed promise, but more research on these models is needed.

Veterans have access to their medical records through the VA's My HealtheVet system (VA, 2012i). Furthermore, they can download their medical records and read, print, or save them to a computer using the Blue Button program (VA, 2012b). Veterans can self-enter several types of information in My HealtheVet, including personal health indicators (such as blood pressure, weight, and heart rate), emergency contact information, names of health care providers, laboratory test results, family health history,

BOX 7-1
Department of Veterans Affairs (VA) Health Care Enrollment
Priority Groups

Group 1: Veterans with VA-rated service-connected disabilities 50% or more disabling; and veterans determined by VA to be unemployable due to service-connected conditions.

Group 2: Veterans with VA-rated service-connected disabilities 30% or 40% disabling.

Group 3: Veterans who are Former Prisoners of War (FPOWs); veterans awarded a Purple Heart medal; veterans whose discharge was for a disability that was incurred or aggravated in the line of duty; veterans with VA-rated service-connected disabilities 10% or 20% disabling; veterans awarded special eligibility classification under Title 38, U.S.C. § 1151, "benefits for individuals disabled by treatment or vocational rehabilitation"; and veterans awarded the Medal of Honor.

Group 4: Veterans who are receiving aid and attendance or housebound benefits from VA; and veterans who have been determined by VA to be catastrophically disabled.

Group 5: Non-service-connected veterans and noncompensable service-connected veterans rated 0% disabled by VA with annual income and/or net worth below the VA national income threshold and geographically-adjusted income threshold for their resident location; veterans receiving VA pension benefits; and veterans eligible for Medicaid programs.

Group 6: World War I veterans; Compensable 0% service-connected veterans; veterans exposed to ionizing radiation during atmospheric testing or during the occupation of Hiroshima and Nagasaki; Project 112/Shipboard Hazard and Defense (SHAD) participants; veterans exposed to the defoliant Agent Orange while serving in the Republic of Vietnam between 1962 and 1975; veterans of the Gulf War that served between August 2, 1990, and November 11, 1998; veterans who served in a theater of combat operations after November 11, 1998, as follows: (a) currently enrolled veterans and new enrollees who were discharged from active duty on or after January 28, 2003, are eligible for the enhanced benefits for 5-years post-discharge; (b) veterans discharged from active duty before January 28, 2003, who apply for enrollment on or after January 28, 2008, are eligible for this enhanced enrollment benefit through January 27, 2011. *Note:* At the end of this enhanced enrollment priority group placement time period, veterans will be assigned to the highest Priority Group their unique eligibility status at that time qualifies them for.

Group 7: Veterans with gross household income below the geographically adjusted income threshold for their resident location and who agree to pay co-pays.

Group 8: Veterans with gross household income above the VA national income threshold and the geographically adjusted income threshold for their resident location and who agree to pay co-pays.
a. **Veterans eligible for enrollment:** Noncompensable 0% service-connected and: *Subpriority a:* Enrolled as of January 16, 2003, and who have remained enrolled since that date and/or placed in this subpriority due to changed eligibility status; *Subpriority b:* Enrolled on or after June 15, 2009, whose income exceeds the current VA National Income Thresholds or VA National Geographic Income Thresholds by 10% or less.
b. **Veterans eligible for enrollment:** Nonservice-connected and: *Subpriority c:* Enrolled as of January 16, 2003, and who have remained enrolled since that date and/or placed in this subpriority due to changed eligibility status; *Subpriority d:* Enrolled on or after June 15, 2009, whose income exceeds the current VA National Income Thresholds or VA National Geographic Income Thresholds by 10% or less.
c. **Veterans not eligible for enrollment:** Veterans not meeting the criteria above: *Subpriority e:* Noncompensable 0% service-connected; and *Subpriority g:* Nonservice-connected.

SOURCE: VA, 2012f.

and military health history. Military service information, such as service dates and deployment periods, is also included in veterans' records.

Disability Compensation for Undiagnosed Illnesses

The diagnoses that Gulf War veterans receive have a direct effect on their ability to obtain disability compensation. In 1995, compensation for service-connected chronic disabilities due to undiagnosed illnesses was established (38 CFR Sec. 3.317). The original regulation specified that the illness had to be manifested during the Gulf War or during the 2 years after conclusion of service. The regulation was amended three times to extend the manifestation period and clarify the intent of the regulation; the last change was published in 2011 (76 F.R. 250 [December 29, 2011]). In addition to an undiagnosed illness, the regulation allows compensation for a medically unexplained CMI that is defined by a cluster of signs or symptoms.

Because of the complexity of the disability patterns and the law governing Gulf War disability rating policy, VA produced a training letter for regional Veterans Benefits Administration (VBA) personnel, explaining the rules for disability compensation for undiagnosed illness and a medically unexplained CMI (VA, 2010). The letter and additional materials are sent to examiners to explain how to evaluate Gulf War veterans' chronic disabilities more effectively (VA, 2012e). The training letter should eliminate some of the confusion surrounding VA's disability-compensation policy; however, a veteran must receive a qualifying diagnosis before applying for disability compensation.

VA and DOD administer a joint pre-discharge program so that service members can file claims for disability compensation up to 180 days before separation or retirement from military service (VA, 2012c). Three components make up the pre-discharge program: the Benefits Delivery at Discharge program (BDD), Quick Start, and the Integrated Disability Evaluation System (IDES). BDD allows service members to apply for disability compensation from VA before separation or retirement (VA, 2008). To receive VA disability compensation within the goal of 60 days after separation, veterans must submit their claims 60–180 days before release from active duty. The goal of the Quick Start program also is to give service members the opportunity to apply for disability compensation from VA while still on active duty (VA, 2009b). However, unlike the BDD program, it is targeted to service members who have fewer than 60 days remaining on active duty, full-time reserve or National Guard members, and others who do not meet the BDD criteria requiring availability of all evaluations before discharge. The goals of the IDES program are to provide "a single disability exam conducted to VA standards that will be used by both Departments [VA and DOD], a single disability rating completed by VA that is binding upon both Departments, and expeditious payment of VA benefits within 30 days of a service member's separation from service" (Rooney, 2012b; VA, 2012c). The IDES program includes a medical examination, but the program is administrative and independent of clinical care and treatment (Rooney, 2012b). Under the IDES program, the wait time for veterans to receive disability compensation from VA and DOD has decreased from an average of 240 days in 2007 (before implementation of the IDES program) to an average of 50 days in 2012 (Rooney, 2012a).

In 2009, the number of pre–September 2001 Gulf War–era veterans who had service-connected undiagnosed illnesses and received health care through VHA was 18,002, or nearly 0.3% of the total Gulf War–era cohort (VA, 2011d), compared with 2,980 in 2000 and 4,439 in 2005.[3]

Data are available on the numbers of pre–September 2001 Gulf War–era veterans who have been granted disability compensation for their undiagnosed illnesses. In FY 2009, the number was 24,409 (VA, 2011d), and that was substantially higher than in previous years—for example, it was 6,109 in FY 2000 and 7,322 in FY 2005. Because not all veterans receive their health care through VHA, it is not possible to determine whether the veterans who are identified as having an undiagnosed illness in the VHA system overlap with the veterans who are receiving disability compensation through VBA.

VA has estimated that a higher percentage of veterans of the Iraq and Afghanistan wars (about 45%) have applied for disability compensation compared to veterans of the 1991 Gulf War (about 20%) (Hickey, July 18, 2012). The average number of medical conditions claimed by the Iraq and Afghanistan war veterans is 8.5. Information was not found on the categories of medical conditions for which the veterans of the Iraq and Afghanistan wars are receiving disability compensation.

AN APPROACH TO ORGANIZING SERVICES FOR CARE OF VETERANS WHO HAVE CHRONIC MULTISYMPTOM ILLNESS

As noted above, VA, in conjunction with DOD, has already committed in principle to expeditious completion of a disability examination for soldiers who are leaving active duty (Rooney, 2012b; VA, 2012c). However, the disability examination process is independent of clinical care and treatment. A PACT team will be incapable of properly managing a veteran who

---

[3]VA (2011b) defines an undiagnosed illness as "a chronic disability which manifested either during active military, naval, or air service in the Southwest Asia theater of operations during the Gulf War, or to a degree of 10 percent or more not later than December 31, 2011. Additionally, the disability cannot be attributed to any known clinical diagnosis by history, physical examination, and laboratory tests."

has CMI or any of its common comorbidities without a comprehensive health assessment and without a definitive disability determination. A comprehensive health assessment is a prerequisite for producing a comprehensive personal care plan, for engaging the patient as a partner in managing the care plan, and for determining the resources that will be needed for the particular veteran's team to execute the care plan. It is patently impossible to accomplish that in the context of a PACT clinic under ordinary operating conditions. In the absence of a comprehensive health assessment, a veteran who has CMI cannot receive high-quality care. With respect to the disability determination, maximum symptom resolution and functional capacity cannot be reached until pending disability dispositions are resolved. Disability is a fluid phenomenon and must be reassessed periodically, but this is not an acceptable argument for deferring disability determination beyond the time when a PACT primary care clinician is expected to initiate a comprehensive personal care plan. Thus, without a comprehensive health assessment and a disability determination, a PACT cannot provide an adequate medical home and a veteran cannot get high-quality care.

The postseparation comprehensive health assessment is useful not only for initiating care but for making initial triage decisions. VHA already has in place a basic setup for a stepped care system for veterans who have CMI. Most CMI patients can and should be managed in an ordinary PACT setting with appropriate adjustments as discussed below. In larger settings, such as VAMCs, there may be a sufficient concentration of CMI patients and a sufficient concentration of interested clinicians to justify the development of a dedicated CMI-PACT or CMI clinic days in a particular PACT made up of interested and expert primary care clinicians, behavioral health clinicians, pain specialists, neurologic consultants, physical rehabilitation clinicians, multiple care coordination and measurement-based management resources, patient-education experts, and others as needed. A needs assessment would show what expertise is necessary and what adjustments are necessary in the clinical constitution of the CMI-PACT team. It is known from experience with, for example, pediatric special-needs clinics that a fully adequate concentration of dedicated human resources, functioning well as a team, is expensive but cost-effective in managing patients who have complex conditions (McAllister et al., 2007; Murphy et al., 2011). Disability care coordination organizations, which coordinate care for people with disabilities who often have multiple, complex physical health, mental health, and psychosocial comorbidities, have also demonstrated the effectiveness of a team approach (Mastal et al., 2007; Palsbo and Ho, 2007; Palsbo et al., 2006). A CMI-PACT team might require six or eight full-time-equivalent clinical professionals, or even more, for the comprehensive and orderly management of 1,000 veterans who have active CMI and its associated comorbidities. Such a clinic may be useful as a consultation center for less severely affected patients whose continuing care is managed in more distant, less well resourced PACTS. Perhaps 5–10% of veterans who have CMI might benefit from such a referral. A more extremely affected subset, perhaps 0.5%–1.0%, might need referral to a center of excellence, such as a WRIISC, where deep expertise is available and state-of-the-art modalities are being developed. The criteria for stepping care up to the next level of intensity will generally include difficulty of managing or failure to manage symptoms adequately, but the criteria would be specified, and the transition needs to be managed so that continuity of care is achieved, consistency is maintained, and communication between sites of care is ensured. Many lapses in quality occur during transitions of care to different settings, so VHA should monitor closely and periodically evaluate the adequacy of communication and the coordination of care among settings when care is stepped.

As noted above, most veterans who have CMI can be managed in a PACT, but care in this setting will fail unless the PACT can adjust the visit schedule to accommodate extended, complex visits; access the specific team members and clinical expertise needed to follow the care plan, including nonclinic care and follow-up; and master the implementation strategies necessary to incorporate the multitude of relevant CPGs, to master team-based care, to navigate the delicate territory between team-based care and developing an accountable personal relationship with patients, and to incorporate self-management strategies into the fabric of the personal care plan. VHA has many of those elements already available and ready to be organized into a system that can render excellent care to veterans who have CMI.

Perhaps the most important of those preconditions is VHA's commitment to make the time available to the primary care team to address the multiple issues that these patients are dealing with. No matter how deep and available the expertise of team members and no matter how successfully implementation is carried out, the primary care team will fail unless it has enough time. Studies of somatizing patients have shown that they can consume substantially more resources than those used by comparable patients who are not so afflicted (Bermingham et al., 2010; Burton et al., 2012; Konnopka et al., 2012; Reid et al., 2002). Clinic visits themselves take longer because many symptoms are interacting with one another in unique and ever-changing ways that require frequent adjustments in the care plan. Multiple team members will need time together to integrate their varied expertise into a coherent and internally consistent plan. It takes time to negotiate competing priorities and to set priorities among and sequence interventions, for example, to work out how a course of cognitive behavioral therapy can be fit into a physical rehabilitation program and how to adjust the timing of several medications. Much PACT-based care can be rendered without a visit, by using the telephone, computer, smart telephone, or other modalities; it takes time to plan, record, communicate, and integrate a care plan that is executed through these modalities. And it takes time to learn to function as a team, to maintain team-based care skills, and to meet together as a team to assign responsibilities for elements of the plan.

VHA can be viewed as the largest health education and health professional training institution in the nation, and it has active interprofessional team training programs in palliative care and geriatrics; it has recently extended interprofessional team-based training into a small number of primary care settings (VA, 2011f). VHA has begun routinely incorporating behavioral health and complementary medicine professionals into PACT teams, as have DOD and civilian patient-centered medical homes (PCMHs). Those laudable efforts should be dramatically expanded so that all PACTs consist of teams whose members have been systematically trained to work together and are given time to do so. Preclinic huddles, team meetings to hammer out complex care plans, joint interprofessional training, communication to consolidate the multiple "touches" that various team members have made in executing a care plan, and, above all, time dedicated to developing and maintaining healthy team dynamics are prerequisites of successful team-based care. Such an investment will pay more than it costs in reduced hospitalizations, emergency department visits, consultant charges, and diagnostic testing. An occasional averted hospitalization will buy a year's worth of care management and behavioral health consultation.

The Institute for Healthcare Improvement (IHI) breakthrough collaborative series offers a useful model for promoting and maintaining organizational change from a continuous quality-improvement perspective by facilitating the emergence of a "learning network." A continuous quality-improvement approach communicates that change is continuous and sustained and provides evidence about the degree of change within the organization. IHI has recommended the Plan Do Study Act (PDSA) cycle with specific and clear goals for changing practices and assessing whether a change is an improvement (see Figure 7-1). The approach also acknowledges that change and improvement are not immediate or one-shot and that they take time. The idea that mistakes can be identified and corrected is built into the cycle. Continuous quality improvement also allows for incorporation of new models of care, such as integrative medicine and optimal healing environments, into the PACT care process when they are needed (IOM, 2009; Jonas and Chez, 2004). Periodic program evaluation is essential to determine whether the process put onto paper and disseminated throughout VHA is being applied (Walter et al., 2010).

VA clinicians have already demonstrated the capacity to use PDSA methods for quality improvement. The model should be applied to the care of patients who have CMI.

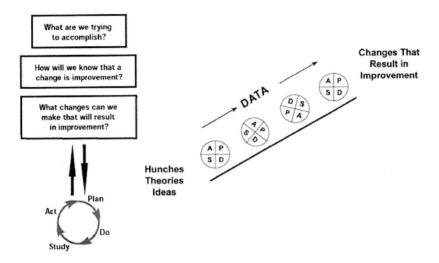

FIGURE 7-1 Institute for Healthcare Improvement Plan Do Study Act model. SOURCE: Reproduced with permission from IHI (Institute for Healthcare Improvement).

Dissemination and implementation of new guidelines require a long-term perspective and the creation of a clinical-care environment in which continuous change in systems of care is the norm. Organizational-level change demands changes in procedures or systems, active communication and marketing of innovation, training, measurement and monitoring, and engagement of key stakeholders (Ruzek and Rosen, 2009).

Implementation science is an emerging field; it is turning out to be highly technical and surprisingly distinct from clinical science in its methods and outcomes. Implementation of multiple guidelines for management of chronic conditions is difficult, requiring complex teamwork by staff who are otherwise fully engaged in caring for patients in distress. Successful implementation has its own measures of success that are distinct from clinical outcomes. It is difficult to implement change in clinics that are highly stressed, that are seriously understaffed, or that operate under rigid directives that discourage flexible problem solving. Successful implementation is a highly local process—best practices do not all look the same—that requires an accurate appraisal of initial conditions and the application of active problem-solving skills. For example, one clinic may reprogram an appointment clerk to become the telephone-based part of the care-management system, and another may be able to use a dedicated care manager for this task. At the heart of successful implementation is the capacity to find workarounds; to sequence elements according to local strengths, opportunities, constraints, and preferences; and especially to address unexpected difficulties and unintended consequences. It is also necessary to collect data systematically on processes of care, on how to effect process change when necessary, on the results of changes with respect to intermediate outcomes, on what works and what does not, and on unintended consequences of changes. The implementation team must be prepared not only to collect information but to reflect on its implications and to act on it with the next process-adjustment cycle. Practice redesign requires a series of linked incremental steps—it is not accomplished in one step. The PDSA method described above has been used successfully in a variety of primary care settings to improve practice.

Implementation work that uses the PDSA method has a unique approach. If changes in disease-specific outcomes are used as the principal measure of success, valuable progress can occur. The road to improved disease state is long and difficult—it is actually many roads—and is beset with so many problems that it requires an approach to dealing with many unexpected problems. Progress needs to be measured by success in solving operational and functional problems that appear one after another, not just in improved disease outcomes. An improved disease state will appear only after a long run of successful interim problem-solving steps.

Many primary care practice redesign organizations (such as TransforMed, HealthTeamWorks, and the Institute for Clinical Systems Improvement) have learned that practice coaches are highly useful (or indispensable) to practices as they begin their redesign efforts. Thus, implementation teams should include health coaches, integrative-medicine practitioners, and other local practice resources that can help practices to work out local changes and solutions to the problem of implementing multiple CPGs for their own unique patient-panel demands under variable local conditions.

The value of learning collaboratives or learning communities must be stressed. Practices, coaches, and other forms of technical support are valuable, but local practice teams often benefit most from the experience of their peers in similar circumstances, and periodic meetings in which ideas and solutions can be exchanged will pay handsome dividends.

Thus, implementation success depends on teams that work well together, that practice active creative problem solving, that maintain flexibility, and that persist in the face of failure—that demonstrate resilience, the ability to learn and improve. Progress toward complete implementation of a guideline is measured in terms of successfully solving one after another the small problems that arise in the course of PDSA work. Use of metrics can lead to improved care and ultimately lead to healthier patients and better outcomes.

A practice that is ready for successful redesign cannot be understood by looking only at workflow; it must also be assessed for active, flexible problem solving. Over time, such a practice can be expected to have shaped workflow to solve the problems of the particular patients in the panel with the particular resources at hand.

SELECT MODELS OF CARE USED BY OTHER ORGANIZATIONS

As noted above, most veterans receive some of or all their care outside the VHA system of clinics in the civilian sector. Civilian settings are more variable and generally less well resourced, and their clinicians are generally less able to devote the time needed to manage CMI and its attendant comorbidities properly in the context of a busy daily practice. Stepped care is much harder in the civilian setting, because specialty resources are less available. Perhaps most important, primary care clinicians in the civilian setting are less familiar with the characteristics of CMI in veteran populations and therefore less adept at creating the complex personal care plans described above. Nevertheless, PCMHs are rapidly appearing in this sector, and the practice-redesign efforts necessary to produce PCMHs will benefit veterans who have CMI and are seeking care—particularly if VHA can extend its resources to these practices. A civilian PCMH that is rendering care to veterans who have CMI would benefit from the following:

- Notification from VHA of the names, disability status, comprehensive health assessment, and other medical care records of the veterans under care, as allowed under the Health Insurance Portability and Accountability Act.
- VHA CPGs applicable to the specific patients, particularly those related to time allocations and team expertise.
- Recommended care-team membership for the patients.
- Access, via telehealth or other ECHO-like variations, to specific team members who have the expertise necessary for the management of the patients, such as neurologists adept at managing traumatic brain injury or acupuncturists adept at pain management.
- Access to consultation with or referral to VAMCs, WRIISCs, and other resources that may benefit veterans as specific problems arise that cannot be managed adequately in the civilian PCMH.

DISSEMINATING EVIDENCE-BASED GUIDELINES THROUGH THE DEPARTMENT OF VETERANS AFFAIRS SYSTEM

The flow of evidence-based information (EBI)—knowledge transfer—through a system to influence policy and practice has become a major topic of focus in the era of evidence-based medicine. It is particularly important when the sheer volume of research data appears to have only slight influence on clinician-practice behaviors. As a result, research has shifted attention from mere generation of guidelines to concerns about their dissemination and implementation (Grimshaw and Russell, 1993; Thomas et al., 1999). Knowledge transfer, some suggest, may occur in three stages: diffusion, dissemination, and implementation (Lomas, 1993). The stages are characterized by increasing specificity, targeting, and customization, leading, in theory, to the adoption of new information that changes practice and policy. Successful models of knowledge transfer do not yet exist (French et al., 2012), but recent work is offering some useful insights into the processes that potentially would help in disseminating EBI, such as practice guidelines. It is instructive to elucidate the three stages and the distinctions among them before discussing the relevance of knowledge transfer in treating for CMI by clinicians in the VA health system.

Diffusion is a passive process that involves spread of EBI with little attention to specificity in defining the target audience or to the customization of the information itself. Publication of studies in professional journals or coverage of scientific studies in the mass media may garner a widespread audience for the message (Viswanath et al., 2008) but may or may not attract the attention of clinicians and patients unless they are already attuned to the topic. Although print media may remain an important source for some physicians and patients, few physicians read medical journals for the latest scientific findings, given the sheer amount of published literature, busy schedules, and possible lack of suitability in how the information is presented (Lomas, 1993; Thomas et al., 1999). Patient-related factors may also act as barriers to using EBI (Thomas et al., 1999).

Dissemination is more deliberate flow of information toward a defined target audience, and the information itself is more customized. Examples include evidence reviews, practice guidelines, and consensus statements.

Implementation goes beyond reaching the intended audience, clinicians. The new information is actually used to change practice behaviors. Given its more ambitious goal, implementation is facilitated by a sharper focus on addressing organizational barriers to the adoption of EBI (Ramanadhan et al., 2012). Localization and customization of EBI will go a long way in facilitating implementation. Appropriate incentives and sanctions may help in this phase. Implementation of guidelines for treatment of veterans who have CMI was discussed in detail earlier in this chapter.

Channels or sources on which physicians rely for EBI, the nature of the information and messages that appeal to them, and the conditions that improve or hinder their capacity to use EBI define the target audience and guide the methods used to approach them. Diffusion and dissemination, in theory, could create awareness about new developments or consensus guidelines but do not necessarily address the day-to-day reality of the clinicians in VHA. They are, however, critical in creating the necessary "readiness for change" in practice behaviors. Change in practice behaviors requires "enabling factors" that address barriers that deter implementation (Lomas, 1993). Behavior change is most likely when environmental changes accompany dissemination of EBI. System changes and support systems will also reinforce changed practice behaviors and may enable their maintenance.

CLINICIANS' BEHAVIOR CHANGE: SYSTEM AND INTERPERSONAL DETERMINANTS

The role of clinicians is critical in any adoption of health care innovations, and much of the adoption and maintenance of innovations requires change in clinicians' behaviors (Gunter and Whittal, 2010). The literature of a variety of fields—including communication, sociology, marketing, psychology, and business—offers useful pointers to understanding how practice behaviors could potentially be changed.

- Peer networks, such as the learning communities described above, have a profound influence on adoption of new behaviors and skills (Bernstein et al., 2009; IOM, 2012; Ramanadhan et al., 2010). Peers could potentially introduce new information, norms, and skills in a network and thereby facilitate the adoption of EBI. Some peers could model new behaviors and skills, making learning of new skills smoother. A network of peers in which communication and informal transfer are routine may lead to the emergence of "learning organizations" in which acquisition of new information, skills, and behaviors can be made routine.
- Opinion leaders and champions, particularly in local health centers, may carry considerable weight in the community of clinicians, facilitating behavior changes and making adoption of new practices acceptable (Moore et al., 2004). One study of knowledge transfer of evidence-based technology that included screening, brief intervention, and referral to treatment conducted in emergency departments found that having local staff as champions made a big difference in adoption and maintenance of a new practice (Bernstein et al., 2009).
- The role of leadership is critical in overcoming barriers to implementation as it ensures quality control, endorsement, priority setting, and the creation of an overall climate of innovation support (Yano et al., 2012).
- Behaviors that are substantive departures from existing practices could be more difficult to change; in a similar vein, complex interventions in contrast to simpler interventions are difficult to imple-

ment and less likely to be adopted (McGovern et al., 2004; Rogers, 1995).

- Organizational constraints—such as inflexible rules, lack of incentives, and potential for negative sanctions—can deter EBI-based changes in practice.
- New methods for connecting EBI to practice, such as appropriate methodology, could link evidence to practices better in the context of the reality of clinical variation.

The advent of information and communication technologies has enabled the development of decision-support systems that facilitate the adoption of recommendations. Decision-support systems, particularly ones that draw on such electronic health records as those used by VA, may provide patient-specific information to a clinician when needed in a manner that is user-friendly. These systems are especially effective when they are user-friendly, easily available, and part of a physician's work flow (Thomas et al., 1999). Thomas et al. (1999) argued that such design considerations as easier navigation, clear indexing, and forgiving interfaces enhance the utility of communication technologies to facilitate behavior change.

As asserted earlier, customization is a critical element in facilitating adoption of innovations. A recommended innovation should be flexible, easy to try out, and customizable to local conditions, and it should have some advantage over current practices (Rogers, 1995). Customization demands careful audience segmentation and designing of intervention components that meet the needs of segments of the audience. In one study, VA tried a social marketing approach to disseminate a new model of collaborative care to treat depression (Luck et al., 2009). In the model, the intervention targeted not just the physicians but other staff, such as local leaders, frontline staff, and managers; it focused on cultural change in the larger organization. Marketing was also reported to be a critical determinant in the national dissemination of a new model to promote collaborative care for depression in the VA system (Smith et al., 2008). Those efforts, in theory, reduce resistance from people in an organization to adopt innovations and ease the change in clinician behaviors.

SUMMARY

VHA faces extraordinary challenges in caring for the burgeoning population of veterans who have CMI. It is possible to meet the challenges with adequate clinician education and support, organization and preparation of care teams that fit the needs of the veterans, establishment of implementation protocols that lead to continuous quality improvement, dissemination of these successes to other clinical teams and settings that are struggling with similar problems, and extension of VHA resources to civilian settings, where most veterans receive their care.

REFERENCES

Arora, S., S. Kalishman, D. Dion, D. Som, K. Thornton, A. Bankhurst, J. Boyle, M. Harkins, K. Moseley, G. Murata, M. Komaramy, J. Katzman, K. Colleran, P. Deming, and S. Yutzy. 2011. Partnering urban academic medical centers and rural primary care clinicians to provide complex chronic disease care. *Health Affairs* 30(6):1176-1184.

Bermingham, S. L., A. Cohen, J. Hague, and M. Parsonage. 2010. The cost of somatisation among the working-age population in England for the year 2008-2009. *Mental Health in Family Medicine* 7(2):71-84.

Bernstein, E., D. Topp, E. Shaw, C. Girard, K. Pressman, E. Woolcock, and J. Bernstein. 2009. A preliminary report of knowledge translation: Lessons from taking screening and brief intervention techniques from the research setting into regional systems of care. *Academic Emergency Medicine* 16(11):1225-1233.

Budzi, D., S. Lurie, K. Singh, and R. Hooker. 2010. Veterans' perceptions of care by nurse practitioners, physician assistants, and physicians: A comparison from satisfaction surveys. *Journal of the American Academy of Nurse Practitioners* 22(3):170-176.

Burton, C., K. McGorm, G. Richardson, D. Weller, and M. Sharpe. 2012. Healthcare costs incurred by patients repeatedly referred to secondary medical care with medically unexplained symptoms: A cost of illness study. *Journal of Psychosomatic Research* 72(3):242-247.

Chou, R., A. Qaseem, V. Snow, D. Casey, J. T. Cross Jr., P. Shekelle, and D. K. Owens. 2007. Diagnosis and treatment of low back pain: A joint clinical practice guideline from the American College of Physicians and the American Pain Society. *Annals of Internal Medicine* 147:478-491.

French, S. D., S. E. Green, D. A. O'Connor, J. E. McKenzie, J. J. Francis, S. Michie, R. Buchbinder, P. Schattner, N. Spike, and J. M. Grimshaw. 2012. Developing theory-informed behaviour change interventions to implement evidence into practice: A systematic approach using the theoretical domains framework. *Implementation Science* 7(38).

Furey, P. 2012 (unpublished). *Analysis of the Social Media Discussion of Chronic Multi-Symptom Illness in Veterans of the Iraq and Afghanistan Wars*. Analysis commissioned by the Committee on Gulf War and Health: Treatment of Chronic Multisymptom Illness, Institute of Medicine, Washington, DC.

Gibson, T. B., T. A. Lee, C. S. Vogeli, J. Hidalgo, G. S. Carls, K. Sredl, S. DesHarnais, W. D. Marder, K. B. Weiss, T. V. Williams, and A. E. Shields. 2009. A four-system comparison of patients with chronic illness: The military health system, Veterans Health Administration, Medicaid, and commercial plans. *Military Medicine* 174(9):936-943.

Grimshaw, J. M., and I. T. Russell. 1993. Effect of clinical guidelines on medical practice: A systematic review of rigorous evaluations. *Lancet* 342(8883):1317-1322.

Gunter, R. W., and M. L. Whittal. 2010. Dissemination of cognitive-behavioral treatments for anxiety disorders: Overcoming barriers and improving patient access. *Clinical Psychology Review* 30(2):194-202.

Harada, N. D., V. M. Villa, and R. Andersen. 2002. Satisfaction with VA and non-VA outpatient care among veterans. *American Journal of Medical Quality* 17(4):155-164.

Hickey, A. A. 2012 (July 18). Statement of Allison A. Hickey, Under Secretary for Benefits, Veterans Benefits Administration (VBA), U.S. Department of Veterans Affairs (VA). In *House Committee on Oversight and Government Reform, Subcommittee on National Security, Homeland Defense, and Foreign Operations*. http://oversight.house.gov/wp-content/uploads/2012/07/7-18-12-Hickey-Testimony.pdf (accessed September 29, 2012).

Hunt, S. C. 2012 (unpublished). *VA Approaches to the Management of Chronic Multi-Symptom Illness in Gulf War I Veterans.* Presentation at the Third Committee Meeting, April 12, 2012, Irvine, CA.

Hynes, D. M., K. Koelling, K. Stroupe, N. Arnold, K. Mallin, M. W. Sohn, F. M. Weaver, L. Manheim, and L. Kok. 2007. Veterans' access to and use of Medicare and Veterans Affairs health care. *Medical Care* 45(3):214-223.

IOM (Institute of Medicine). 2009. *Integrative Medicine and the Health of the Public: A Summary of the February 2009 Summit.* Washington, DC: The National Academies Press.

IOM. 2012. *Best Care at Lower Cost: The Path to Continuously Learning Health Care in America.* Washington, DC: The National Academies Press.

Jonas, W. B., and R. A. Chez. 2004. Toward optimal healing environments in health care. *Journal of Alternative and Complementary Medicine* 10:S1-S6.

Katzman, J. 2012. Making connections: Using telehealth to improve the diagnosis and treatment of complex regional pain syndrome, an underrecognized neuroinflammatory disorder. *Journal of Neuroimmune Pharmacology.* Published online October 2, 2012.

Kehle, S. M., N. Greer, I. Rutks, and T. J. Wilt. 2011. *Interventions to Improve Veterans' Access to Care: A Systematic Review of the Literature.* Health Services Research & Development Service, Department of Veterans Affairs, Washington, DC.

Konnopka, A., R. Schaefert, S. Heinrich, C. Kaufmann, M. Luppa, W. Herzog, and H. H. Konig. 2012. Economics of medically unexplained symptoms: A systematic review of the literature. *Psychotherapy & Psychosomatics* 81(5):265-275.

Lincoln, A. E., D. A. Helmer, A. I. Schneiderman, M. Li, H. Copeland, M. K. Prisco, M. T. Wallin, H. K. Kang, and B. H. Natelson. 2006. The war-related illness and injury study centers: A resource for deployment-related health concerns. *Military Medicine* 171(7):577-585.

Lomas, J. 1993. Diffusion, dissemination, and implementation: Who should do what? *Annals of the New York Academy of Sciences* 703:226-237.

Luck, J., F. Hagigi, L. E. Parker, E. M. Yano, L. V. Rubenstein, and J. E. Kirchner. 2009. A social marketing approach to implementing evidence-based practice in VHA QUERI: The TIDES depression collaborative care model. *Implementation Science* 4:64.

Mastal, M. F., M. E. Reardon, and M. English. 2007. Innovations in disability care coordination organizations: Integrating primary care and behavioral health clinical systems. *Professional Case Management* 12(1):27-36.

McAllister, J. W., E. Presler, and W. C. Cooley. 2007. Practice-based care coordination: A medical home essential. *Pediatrics* 120(3):e723-e733.

McGovern, M. P., T. S. Fox, H. Y. Xie, and R. E. Drake. 2004. A survey of clinical practices and readiness to adopt evidence-based practices: Dissemination research in an addiction treatment system. *Journal of Substance Abuse Treatment* 26(4):305-312.

Moore, K. A., R. H. Peters, H. A. Hills, J. B. LeVasseur, A. R. Rich, W. M. Hunt, M. S. Young, and T. W. Valente. 2004. Characteristics of opinion leaders in substance abuse treatment agencies. *American Journal of Drug and Alcohol Abuse* 30(1):187-203.

Murphy, N. A., P. S. Carbone, Council on Children With Disabilities, and American Academy of Pediatrics. 2011. Parent-provider-community partnerships: Optimizing outcomes for children with disabilities. *Pediatrics* 128(4):795-802.

Nicholas, W., D. O. Farley, M. E. Vaiana, and S. Cretin. 2001. *Putting Practice Guidelines to Work in the Department of Defense Medical System.* Santa Monica, CA: RAND Corporation.

Palsbo, S. E., and P. S. Ho. 2007. Consumer evaluation of a disability care coordination organization. *Journal of Health Care for the Poor and Underserved* 18(4):887-901.

Palsbo, S. E., M. F. Mastal, and L. T. O'Donnell. 2006. Disability care coordination organizations: Improving health and function in people with disabilities. *Lippincott's Case Managment* 11(5):255-264.

Petersen, L. A., M. M. Byrne, C. N. Daw, J. Hasche, B. Reis, and K. Pietz. 2010. Relationship between clinical conditions and use of Veterans Affairs health care among Medicare-enrolled veterans. *Health Services Research* 45(3):762-791.

Petzel, R. A. 2012. What does the future look like for VA healthcare? *U.S. Medicine: the Voice of Federal Medicine*, http://www.usmedicine.com/outlook/what-does-the-future-look-like-for-va-healthcare.html (accessed September 28, 2012).

Ramanadhan, S., J. Weicha, S. Gortmaker, K. M. Emmons, and K. Viswanath. 2010. Informal training in staff networks to support dissemination of health promotion programs. *American Journal of Health Promotion* 25(1):12-18.

Ramanadhan, S., J. Crisostomo, J. Alexander-Molloy, E. Gandelman, M. Grullon, V. Lora, and K. Viswanath. 2012. Perceptions of evidence-based programs among community-based organizations tackling health disparities: A qualitative study. *Health Education Research* 27(4):717-728.

Reid, S., S. Wessely, T. Crayford, and M. Hotopf. 2002. Frequent attenders with medically unexplained symptoms: Service use and costs in secondary care. *British Journal of Psychiatry* 180:248-253.

Reinhard, M. J. 2012 (unpublished). *Complementary and Alternative Medicine (CAM) and Chronic Multi-symptom Illness*. Presentation at the Second Committee Meeting, February 29, 2012, Washington, DC.

Reisinger, H. S., S. C. Hunt, A. L. Burgo-Black, and M. A. Agarwal. 2012. A population approach to mitigating the long-term health effects of combat deployments. *Preventing Chronic Disease* 9:E54.

Ren, X. S., L. Kazis, A. Lee, W. Rogers, and S. Pendergrass. 2001. Health status and satisfaction with health care: A longitudinal study among patients served by the Veterans Health Administration. *American Journal of Medical Quaityl* 16(5):166-173.

Rogers, E. M. 1995. *Diffusion of Innovations*. 4th ed. New York: The Free Press.

Rooney, J. A. 2012a. *Testimony Before the Senate Committee on Veterans Affairs*. Hearing on Seamless Transition: Review of the Integrated Disability Evaluation System. 112th Cong. 2nd Sess. May 23, 2012. http://veterans.senate.gov/hearings.cfm?action=release.display&release_id=5a948325-1c39-4251-81a7-a724f9b58c15 (accessed September 28, 2012).

Rooney, J. A. 2012b. Directive-Type Memorandium (DTM) 11-015—Integrated Disability Evaluation System (IDES). Washington, DC: Department of Defense.

Ruzek, J. I., and R. C. Rosen. 2009. Disseminating evidence-based treatments for PTSD in organizational settings: A high priority focus area. *Behaviour Research and Therapy* 47(11):980-989.

Smith, J. L., J. W. Williams, R. R. Owen, L. V. Rubenstein, and E. Chaney. 2008. Developing a national dissemination plan for collaborative care for depression: QUERI series. *Implementation Science* 3.

Stroupe, K. T., D. M. Hynes, A. Giobbie-Harder, E. Z. Oddone, M. Weinberger, D. J. Reda, and W. G. Henderson. 2005. Patient satisfaction and use of Veterans Affairs versus non–Veterans Affairs healthcare services by veterans. *Medical Care* 43(5):453-460.

Thomas, K. W., C. S. Dayton, and M. W. Peterson. 1999. Evaluation of Internet-based clinical decision support systems. *Journal of Medical Internet Research* 1(2):E6.

Tinetti, M. E., T. R. Fried, and C. M. Boyd. 2012. Designing health care for the most common chronic condition–multimorbidity. *Journal of the American Medical Association* 307(23):2493-2494.

VA (Department of Veterans Affairs). 2008. *Benefits Delivery at Discharge (BDD): A Joint VA-DOD Initiative.* VA Pamphlet 21-08-1.

VA. 2009a. *Controlled Breathing Techniques.* War Related Illness and Injury Study Center. Palo Alto, CA.

VA. 2009b. *Quick Start.* http://www.vba.va.gov/predischarge/quickstart.htm (accessed September 29, 2012).

VA. 2009c. *Self-Management: Giving Veteran Patients Tools to Take Control of Their Own Health—A Resource for Health Care Providers.* War Related Illness and Injury Study Center. East Orange, NJ.

VA. 2010 (unpublished). *Training letter 10-01: Adjudicating Claims Based on Service in the Gulf War and Southwest Asia.* http://www.ngwrc.org/docs/VAtl10-01.pdf (accessed September 28, 2012).

VA. 2011a. *Caring for Gulf War I Veterans.* http://www.publichealth.va.gov/docs/vhi/caring-for-gulf-war-veterans-vhi.pdf (accessed March 11, 2013).

VA. 2011b. *Complementary and Integrative Medicine: A Resouce for Veterans, Service Members and Their Families.* War Related Illness and Injury Study Center. East Orange, NJ.

VA. 2011c. *Excercise to Help Manage Chronic Pain and/or Fatigue: A Resource for Veterans, Service Members, and Their Families.* War Related Illness and Injury Study Center. East Orange, NJ.

VA. 2011d. *Gulf War Era Veterans Report: Pre-9/11 (August 2, 1990 to September 10, 2001).* Washington, DC: Department of Veterans Affairs. http://www.va.gov/vetdata/docs/SpecialReports/GW_Pre911_report.pdf (accessed September 28, 2012).

VA. 2011e. *Medically Unexplained Symptoms: A Resource for Veterans, Service Members, and Their Families.* War Related Illness and Injury Study Center. East Orange, NJ.

VA. 2011f. *VA Centers of Excellence in Primary Care Education.* http://www.va.gov/oaa/rfp_coe.asp (accessed September 19, 2012).

VA. 2012a. *Analysis of VA Health Care Utilization Among Operation Enduring Freedom (OEF), Operation Iraqi Freedom (OIF), and Operation New Dawn (OND) Veterans.* http://www.publichealth.va.gov/docs/epidemiology/healthcare-utilization-report-fy2012-qtr2.pdf (accessed September 12, 2012).

VA. 2012b. *Blue Button.* http://www.va.gov/BLUEBUTTON/index.asp (accessed October 24, 2012).

VA. 2012c. Chapter 10 transition assistance. In *Federal Benefits for Veterans, Dependents and Survivors.* http://www.va.gov/opa/publications/benefits_book/benefits_chap10.asp (accessed November 29, 2012).

VA. 2012d. *Department of Veterans Affairs Statistics at a Glance.* http://www.va.gov/vetdata/docs/Quickfacts/Stats_at_a_glance_FINAL.pdf (accessed September 19, 2012).

VA. 2012e. *Gulf War Veterans' Illnesses Task Force Report.* http://www.va.gov/opa/publications/2011_GWVI-TF_Report.pdf (accessed September 28, 2012)

VA. 2012f. *Health Benefits Priority Groups Table.* http://www.va.gov/healthbenefits/resources/priority_groups.asp (accessed November 19, 2012).

VA. 2012g. *Health Care: Patient Centered Care.* http://www.va.gov/health/newsfeatures/20120827a.asp (accessed November 19, 2012).

VA. 2012h. *Improving Quality of Care.* http://www.qualityandsafety.va.gov/qualityofcare/improving-quality-of-care.asp (accessed November 19, 2012).

VA. 2012i. *My HealtheVet.* https://www.myhealth.va.gov/index.html (accessed October 24, 2012).

VA. 2012j. *Patient Aligned Care Team (PACT).* http://www.va.gov/primarycare/pcmh/ (accessed September 28, 2012).

VA. 2012k. *Review of Veterans' Access to Mental Health Care.* VA Office of Inspector General, Veterans Health Administration. http://www.va.gov/oig/pubs/VAOIG-12-00900-168.pdf (accessed September 28, 2012).

VA. 2012l. *War Related Illness and Injury Study Center: What We Do.* http://www.warrelatedillness.va.gov/WARRELATEDILLNESS/about-us/what-we-do.asp (accessed September 28, 2012).

VA and DOD (Department of Defense). 2001a. *Clinical Practice Guideline for Post-Deployment Health Evaluation and Management, Version 1.2.* http://www.healthquality.va.gov/pdh/PDH_cpg.pdf (accessed September 28, 2012).

VA and DOD. 2001b. *Clinical Practice Guideline for the Management of Medically Unexplained Symptoms: Chronic Pain and Fatigue.* http://www.healthquality.va.gov/mus/mus_fulltext.pdf (accessed September 28, 2012).

VA and DOD. 2009a. *Clinical Practice Guideline for the Management of Substance Use Disorders (SUD).* http://www.healthquality.va.gov/sud/sud_full_601f.pdf (accessed September 28, 2012).

VA and DOD. 2009b. *Clinical Practice Guideline: Management of Concussion/Mild Traumatic Brain Injury.* http://www.healthquality.va.gov/mtbi/concussion_mtbi_full_1_0.pdf (accessed September 28, 2012).

VA and DOD. 2009c. *Clinical Practice Guideline: Management of Major Depressive Disorder (MDD).* http://www.healthquality.va.gov/MDD_FULL_3c.pdf (accessed September 28, 2012).

VA and DOD. 2010a. *Clinical Practice Guideline For Management of Post-Traumatic Stress.* http://www.healthquality.va.gov/ptsd/PTSD-FULL-2010a.pdf (accessed September 28, 2012).

VA and DOD. 2010b. *Clinical Practice Guideline: Management of Opioid Therapy for Chronic Pain.* http://www.healthquality.va.gov/COT_312_Full-er.pdf (accessed September 28, 2012).

VA and DOD. 2011. *Manual for Facility Clinical Practice Guideline Champions.* https://www.qmo.amedd.army.mil/general_documents/Champion_Manual.pdf (accessed September 28, 2012).

Viswanath, K., K. D. Blake, H. I. Meissner, N. G. Saiontz, C. Mull, C. S. Freeman, B. Hesse, and R. T. Croyle. 2008. Occupational practices and the making of health news: A national survey of US health and medical science journalists. *Journal of Health Communication* 13(8):759-777.

Walter, J., I. D. Coulter, A. Adler, P. D. Bliese, and R. Nicholas. 2010. Program evaluation of total force fitness in the military. *Military Medicine* 175(8):103-109.

Walters, T. 2011 (unpublished). Institute of Medicine Committee on Gulf War and Health: Treatments for Multi-Symptom Illness, December 12, 2011, Washington, DC.

West, A. N., W. B. Weeks, and A. E. Wallace. 2008. Rural veterans and access to high-quality care for high-risk surgeries. *Health Services Research* 43(5):1737-1751.

Wright, S. M., T. Craig, S. Campbell, J. Schaefer, and C. Humble. 2006. Patient satisfaction of female and male users of Veterans Health Administration services. *Journal of General Internal Medicine* 21 (Suppl 3):S26-S32.

Yano, E. M., L. W. Green, K. Glanz, J. Z. Ayanian, B. S. Mittman, V. Chollette, and L. V. Rubenstein. 2012. Implementation and spread of interventions into the multilevel context of routine practice and policy: Implications for the cancer care continuum. *Journal of the National Cancer Institute Monograph* (44):86-99.

8

Recommendations

The committee, drawing on evidence presented in Chapters 2–7, offers recommendations in five categories:

1. Treatments for chronic multisymptom illness (CMI).
2. The Department of Veterans Affairs (VA) health care system as it is related to improving systems of care and the management of care for veterans who have CMI.
3. Dissemination through the VA health care system of information on caring for veterans who have CMI.
4. Improving the collection and quality of data on outcomes and satisfaction of care of veterans who have CMI and are treated in VA health care facilities.
5. Research on diagnosing and treating CMI and on program evaluation.

TREATMENTS FOR CHRONIC MULTISYMPTOM ILLNESS

In Chapter 4, the committee assessed the evidence on treatments for symptoms associated with CMI. The types of treatments included in the assessment were not predetermined by the committee. Rather, all treatments on which there was evidence were evaluated. Both pharmacologic and nonpharmacologic treatments were assessed.

CMI is a complex condition, and it has multiple co-occurring symptoms that vary from person to person. The committee believed that it was necessary to evaluate both integrative treatment approaches and individual interventions. Therefore, the scientific literature was searched broadly and included nontraditional interventions (for example, complementary medicine and alternative medicine) in addition to traditional interventions (for example, pharmaceuticals). A summary of the search strategy can be found in Chapter 3.

Three studies of interventions for the symptoms associated with CMI were conducted in the 1991 Gulf War veteran population. Those studies were included in the assessment with studies conducted in different populations that had a similar constellation of symptoms. The generalizability of studies on nonveterans to veterans is not known.

As described in Chapter 4, the strength of the evidence on each type of intervention was graded as insufficient, low, moderate, or high. Strength of evidence is not equivalent to efficacy or effectiveness of a treatment. Strength of evidence is a measure of confidence in the body of evidence. Efficacy or effectiveness of treatment takes into account the strength of evidence and the net benefit of the treatment to the patients.

Several studies showing high and moderate strength of evidence were conducted in the 1991 Gulf War veteran population (Donta et al., 2003, 2004; Guarino et al., 2001; Mori et al., 2006). Although the study of doxycycline was found to have high strength of evidence and was conducted in a group of 1991 Gulf War veterans who had CMI, it did not demonstrate efficacy; that is, doxycycline did not reduce or eliminate the symptoms of CMI in the study population (Donta et al., 2004). Of the studies found to have moderate strength of evidence were studies of exercise and group cognitive behavioral therapy (CBT) that were conducted in 1991 Gulf War veterans who had CMI and demonstrated a net benefit in reducing the symptoms associated with CMI (Donta et al., 2003; Guarino et al., 2001; Mori et al., 2006). Those studies evaluated the effects of exercise and CBT in combination and individually. The therapeutic benefit of exercise was unclear in those studies. Group CBT rather than exercise may confer the main therapeutic benefit with respect to physical symptoms. Additional studies, not conducted in 1991 Gulf War veterans, also reported a net benefit of exercise or group CBT in reducing symptoms associated with CMI (Bleichhardt et al., 2004; Lidbeck, 2003; Martin et al., 2007; Peters et al., 2002; Rief et al., 2002; Zaby et al., 2008).

Studies of individual CBT (high strength of evidence) and St. John's wort (SJW; moderate strength of evidence) did not include 1991 Gulf War veterans who had CMI. Studies of individual CBT showed a consistent pattern of symptom improvement in people who had unexplained symptoms (Allen et al., 2006; Escobar et al., 2007; Sharpe et al., 2011; Sumathipala et al., 2000, 2008). Studies of SJW in people who had somatoform disorders also demonstrated symptom improvement (Muller et al., 2004; Volz et al., 2002).

Many symptoms that define CMI are shared with symptoms associated with other conditions: fibromyaliga, chronic pain, chronic fatigue syndrome, somatic symptom disorders, sleep disorders, IBS, functional dyspepsia, depression, anxiety, posttraumatic stress disorder, traumatic brain injury, substance-use and addictive disorders, and self-harm. Therefore, the committee identified guidelines and systematic reviews of treatments for the related and comorbid conditions to determine whether any treatments found to be effective for one of the conditions may be beneficial for CMI. Three pharmaceuticals—selective serotonin reuptake inhibitors (SSRIs), serotonin–norepinephrine reuptake inhibitors (SNRIs), and tricyclic medications—and CBT were found to be effective in managing the majority of the related and comorbid conditions assessed. Many other treatments, both pharmacologic and nonpharmacologic, have also been shown to be effective in managing at least some of the symptoms associated with conditions related to and comorbid with CMI (see Table 5-3).

The best available evidence from studies of treatment for symptoms of CMI and related and comorbid conditions demonstrates that many veterans who have CMI may show some benefit from such medications as SSRIs and SNRIs and from CBT. On the basis of the evidence reviewed, the committee cannot recommend any specific therapy as a set treatment for veterans who have CMI. The committee believes that a "one-size-fits-all" approach is not effective for managing veterans who have CMI and that individualized health care management plans are necessary. The condition is complex and not well understood, and it will require more than simply treating veterans according to a set protocol.

Recommendation 8-1. The Department of Veterans Affairs should implement a systemwide, integrated, multimodal, long-term management approach to manage veterans who have chronic multisymptom illness.

VA already has several programs that could be used to manage veterans who have CMI, such as postdeployment patient-aligned care teams (PD-PACTs), specialty care access networks-extension for community health care outcomes (SCAN-ECHO), and war-related illness and injury study centers (WRIISCs). However, the programs have not been consistently implemented throughout the VA health care system, and they have not been adequately evaluated to learn about their strengths and weaknesses so that changes can be made to improve the quality of care. The committee offers additional recommendations to VA related to making better use of existing programs to manage the care of veterans who have CMI.

IMPROVING CARE OF VETERANS WHO HAVE
CHRONIC MULTISYMPTOM ILLNESS

The first step in providing care of veterans who have CMI is to identify them and bring them into the VA health care system. Prior to separation from the military, VA, in conjunction with the Department of Defense, offers soldiers a disability examination. However, the disability examination is independent of clinical care and treatment. A comprehensive health evaluation, ideally conducted shortly after separation, is important to identify veterans who have CMI, as defined by the committee in Chapter 2, so that they can receive proper care for their CMI and any common comorbidities.

> **Recommendation 8-2. The Department of Veterans Affairs (VA) should commit the necessary resources to ensure that veterans complete a comprehensive health examination immediately upon separation from active duty. The results should become part of a veteran's health record and should be made available to every clinician caring for the veteran, whether in or outside the VA health care system. Coordination of care, focused on transition in care, is essential for all veterans to ensure quality, patient safety, and the best health outcomes. Any veteran who has chronic multisymptom illness should be able to complete a comprehensive health examination.**

> **Recommendation 8-3. The Department of Veterans Affairs should include in its electronic health record a "pop-up" screen to prompt clinicians to ask questions about whether a patient has symptoms consistent with the committee's definition of chronic multisymptom illness.**

Once a veteran has been identified as having CMI and has entered the VA health care system, the next step is to provide comprehensive care for the veteran, not only for CMI but also for any comorbid conditions. VA has developed multiple clinical practice guidelines (CPGs) for medically unexplained symptoms (VA and DOD, 2001b), common comorbidities and conditions with shared symptoms, such as major depressive disorder, posttraumatic stress disorder, traumatic brain injury, and chronic pain (Chou et al., 2007; VA and DOD, 2009a,b,c, 2010a,b), and post-deployment health (VA and DoD, 2001a). However, there is anecdotal evidence that simply adhering to multiple CPGs often is not effective for managing chronic conditions with multiple morbidities such as CMI and can result in incomplete care and decrease patient satisfaction, and increase the likelihood of over-treatment and adverse side effects. As described in Chapter 7, management of the health of veterans who have CMI requires a unique personal care plan for each veteran.

Coordination of care for veterans who have CMI among clinicians and others involved in providing care is essential. VA's PD-PACTs should be able to provide care for veterans who have CMI if properly implemented. The goal of the PD-PACT model is to provide comprehensive, integrated care, including follow-up health care and education (Reisinger et al., 2012). The PD-PACT serves as a veteran's medical home within the VA and uses a team approach to providing care. Team members can include a project manager, primary care clinicians, nurse care managers, mental health clinicians, social workers, and other specialists as needed. The move to a medical home model of care is relatively recent in VA's health care system, and implementation is ongoing (Reisinger et al., 2012).

> **Recommendation 8-4.** The Department of Veterans Affairs (VA) should develop patient-aligned care teams (PACTs) specifically for veterans who have chronic multisymptom illness (CMI; that is, CMI-PACTs) or CMI clinic days in existing PACTs at larger facilities, such as VA medical centers. A needs assessment should be conducted to determine what expertise is necessary to include in a CMI-PACT.

> **Recommendation 8-5.** The Department of Veterans Affairs should commit the resources needed to ensure that patient-aligned care teams have the time and skills required to meet the needs of veterans who have chronic multisymptom illness as specified in the veterans' integrated personal care plans, that the adequacy of time for clinical encounters is measured routinely, and that clinical caseloads are adjusted in response to the data generated by measurements. Data from patient experience-of-care surveys are essential to assist in determining needed adjustments.

> **Recommendation 8-6.** The Department of Veterans Affairs should use patient-aligned care teams (PACTs) that have been demonstrated to be centers of excellence as examples so that other PACTs can build on their experiences.

To address the challenges of bringing care to veterans who lack easy access to VA medical centers, VA adopted the SCAN-ECHO model in 2010. SCAN-ECHO programs are being developed to bring specialty care to veterans who live in rural and other underserved areas. The SCAN-ECHO programs work by connecting clinicians who have expertise in particular specialties through video technology to provide case-based consultation and didactics to isolated primary care clinicians, who would otherwise not have access to care for their patients (Arora et al., 2011). After an initial in-person orientation, the team meets weekly via videoconference to present and discuss patients, and together formulate care plans.

Another VA program is the WRIISC program, which was established in 2001 to serve combat veterans with unexplained illnesses. Veterans are generally referred to a WRIISC (there are three nationwide) by their clinicians when they are not improving and further local expertise is not available (Reinhard, 2012). Veterans in WRIISCs are evaluated by a multidisciplinary team that conducts a comprehensive health assessment and formulates a comprehensive personal care plan aimed at managing symptoms and improving functional health, which is implemented at the WRIISC and given to the referring clinicians (Lincoln et al., 2006). Although WRIISCs have been in place for more than a decade, the committee does not have information on awareness of the program among the teams of professionals caring for veterans who have CMI or among the veterans themselves. Information also is lacking on the effectiveness of the program.

> **Recommendation 8-7. The Department of Veterans Affairs (VA) should develop a process for evaluating awareness among teams of professionals and veterans of its programs for managing veterans who have chronic multisymptom illness, including patient-aligned care teams (PACTs), specialty care access networks (SCANs), and war-related illness and injury study centers (WRIISCs); for providing education where necessary; and for measuring outcomes to determine whether the programs have been successfully implemented and are improving care. Furthermore, VA should take steps to improve coordination of care among PACTs, SCANs, and WRIISCs so that veterans can transition smoothly across these programs.**

DISSEMINATION OF INFORMATION

Many opportunities exist for VA to disseminate information about CMI to clinicians. A major determinant of VA's ability to manage veterans who have CMI is the training of clinicians and teams of professionals in providing care for these patients. Although clinicians are appreciative of the challenges faced by veterans who have CMI and of their suffering, they also are wary of the difficulties in treating these patients (Aiarzaguena et al., 2009). Training clinicians to effectively communicate with and provide care for veterans who have CMI is essential. As noted in Chapter 7, VA can be viewed as the largest health education and health professional training institution in the nation. It has active interprofessional team training programs in palliative care and geriatrics and has recently extended interprofessional team-based training into a small number of primary care settings (VA, 2011). Future training programs for clinicians and other team members caring for veterans who have CMI can be built upon the infrastructure already in place at VA.

> Recommendation 8-8. The Department of Veterans Affairs (VA) should provide resources for and designate "chronic multisymptom illness champions" at each VA medical center. The champions should be integrated into the care system (for example, the patient-aligned care teams) to ensure clear communication and coordination among clinicians.

The champions should be incentivized (for example, by professional advancement and recognition and value-based payment), be given adequate time for office visits with patients who have CMI, have knowledge about the array of therapeutic options that might be useful for treating symptoms associated with CMI, have ready access to a team of other clinicians for consultation, and have training in communication skills. Smaller VA facilities, such as community-based outreach clinics (CBOCs), can benefit from CMI champions. For example, the SCAN-ECHO model can be used so that clinicians in CBOCs or even civilian community-based clinics can contact a CMI champion for expert consultation.

In addition to using CMI champions to train clinicians about CMI, learning networks have been found to be effective tools for disseminating information. Continuous exchange of information among learning networks can lead to improved quality of care. The networks offer a supportive environment for learning skills informally, role models, and a benchmark for an appropriate environment for adopting new guidelines.

> Recommendation 8-9. The Department of Veterans Affairs (VA) should develop learning, or peer, networks to introduce new information, norms, and skills related to managing veterans who have chronic multisymptom illness. Because many veterans receive care outside the VA health care system, clinicians in private practice should be offered the opportunity to be included in the learning networks and VA should have a specific focus on community outreach.

Effective patient–clinician communication and coordination of care are crucial for managing veterans who have CMI and are the foundation of patient-centered care and decision making. They are essential for managing such patients successfully. Chapter 6 outlines factors relating to good patient–clinician interactions and provides recommendations to clinicians to improve their relationships with patients with CMI.

> Recommendation 8-10. The Department of Veterans Affairs should provide required education and training for its clinicians in communi-

cating effectively with and coordinating the care of veterans who have unexplained conditions, such as chronic multisymptom illness.

IMPROVING DATA COLLECTION AND QUALITY

As the committee conducted its assessment of treatments for CMI and of how this condition is managed in the VA health care system, it identified gaps in data on performance. For example, although the WRIISC program has been in place since 2001, the committee did not find a comprehensive evaluation of how well veterans who have been treated through the program are doing or how satisfied they are with their care. What are the measures of success? To assist VA in improving outcomes and ultimately to improve the quality of care that the VA health care system provides, the committee offers the following recommendation.

> **Recommendation 8-11. The Department of Veterans Affairs (VA) should provide the resources needed to expand its data collection efforts to include a national system for the robust capture, aggregation, and analysis of data on the structures, processes, and outcomes of care delivery and on the satisfaction with care among patients who have chronic multisymptom illness so that gaps in clinical care can be evaluated, strategies for improvement can be planned, long-term outcomes of treatment can be assessed, and this information can be disseminated to VA health care facilities.**

Data collection should be derived from structure, process, and outcome measurements. An example of a structure measure is the nurse-to-patient ratio in a health facility. Examples of process measures are the number of veterans were screened for CMI, the total number discharged from the military, and what interventions veterans who have CMI receive. Another process and, also, outcome measure is patient experience-of-care information, which should be collected for both inpatients and outpatients. Patient experience-of-care information should be easily accessible on the Internet and be facility specific. Another example of an outcome measure is the percentage of patients' improvement on a pain scale following an intervention.

RESEARCH RECOMMENDATIONS

This section contains the committee's research recommendations. These recommendations are in two categories, treatments for CMI and research needs related to program evaluation.

Treatments for Chronic Multisymptom Illness

Many of the studies of treatments for CMI reviewed by the committee had methodologic flaws that limited their usefulness for the committee's evaluation.

Recommendation 8-12. Future studies funded and conducted by the Department of Veterans Affairs to assess treatments for chronic multisymptom illness should adhere to the methodologic and reporting guidelines for clinical trials, including appropriate elements (problem–patient–population, intervention, comparison, and outcome of interest) to frame the research question, extended follow-up, active comparators (such as standard-of-care therapies), and consistent, standardized, validated instruments for measuring outcomes.

Examples of methodologic and reporting guidelines include those set forth by such organizations as the Agency for Healthcare Research and Quality and the Institute of Medicine and in such other efforts as the Preferred Reporting Items for Systematic Reviews and Meta-Analyses statement and the Consolidated Standards of Reporting Trials statement.

On the basis of its assessment of the evidence on treatments for CMI, the committee found that several treatments and treatment approaches may be potentially useful for CMI. However, evidence sufficient to support a conclusion on their effectiveness is lacking.

Recommendation 8-13. The Department of Veterans Affairs should fund and conduct studies of interventions that evidence suggests may hold promise for treatment of chronic multisymptom illness. Specific interventions could include biofeedback, acupuncture, St. John's wort, aerobic exercise, motivational interviewing, and multimodal therapies.

Several of the above-mentioned interventions are in the area of complementary and alternative medicine and the VA should consider coordinating future research efforts with the National Institutes of Health's National Center for Complementary and Alternative Medicine.

Program Evaluation

As noted above, the committee did not find comprehensive evaluations of VA programs, such as the PACTs, SCAN-ECHOs programs, and WRIISCs. Program evaluation—including assessments of structures, processes, and outcomes—is essential if VA is to continually improve its services and research.

Recommendation 8-14. The Department of Veterans Affairs (VA) should apply principles of quality and performance improvement to internally evaluate VA programs and research related to treatments for chronic multisymptom illness (CMI) and overall management of veterans who have CMI. This task can be accomplished using such methods as comparative effectiveness research, translational research, implementation science methods, and health systems research.

REFERENCES

Aiarzaguena, J. M., I. Gaminde, G. Grandes, A. Salazar, I. Alonso, and A. Sanchez. 2009. Somatisation in primary care: Experiences of primary care physicians involved in a training program and in a randomised controlled trial. *BMC Family Practice* 10:73.

Allen, L. A., R. L. Woolfolk, J. I. Escobar, M. A. Gara, and R. M. Hamer. 2006. Cognitive-behavioral therapy for somatization disorder: A randomized controlled trial. *Archives of Internal Medicine* 166(14):1512-1518.

Arora, S., S. Kalishman, D. Dion, D. Som, K. Thornton, A. Bankhurst, J. Boyle, M. Harkins, K. Moseley, G. Murata, M. Komaramy, J. Katzman, K. Colleran, P. Deming, and S. Yutzy. 2011. Partnering urban academic medical centers and rural primary care clinicians to provide complex chronic disease care. *Health Affairs* 30(6):1176-1184.

Bleichhardt, G., B. Timmer, and W. Rief. 2004. Cognitive-behavioural therapy for patients with multiple somatoform symptoms: A randomised controlled trial in tertiary care. *Journal of Psychosomatic Research* 56:449-454.

Chou, R., A. Qaseem, V. Snow, D. Casey, J. T. Cross Jr., P. Shekelle, and D. K. Owens. 2007. Diagnosis and treatment of low back pain: A joint clinical practice guideline from the American College of Physicians and the American Pain Society. *Annals of Internal Medicine* 147:478-491.

Donta, S. T., D. J. Clauw, C. C. Engel, Jr., P. Guarino, P. Peduzzi, D. A. Williams, J. S. Skinner, A. Barkhuizen, T. Taylor, L. E. Kazis, S. Sogg, S. C. Hunt, C. M. Dougherty, R. D. Richardson, C. Kunkel, W. Rodriguez, E. Alicea, P. Chiliade, M. Ryan, G. C. Gray, L. Lutwick, D. Norwood, S. Smith, M. Everson, W. Blackburn, W. Martin, J. M. Griffiss, R. Cooper, E. Renner, J. Schmitt, C. McMurtry, M. Thakore, D. Mori, R. Kerns, M. Park, S. Pullman-Mooar, J. Bernstein, P. Hershberger, D. C. Salisbury, J. R. Feussner, and V. A. C. S. S. Group. 2003. Cognitive behavioral therapy and aerobic exercise for Gulf War veterans' illnesses: A randomized controlled trial. *Journal of the American Medical Association* 289(11):1396-1404.

Donta, S. T., C. C. Engel, Jr., J. F. Collins, J. B. Baseman, L. L. Dever, T. Taylor, K. D. Boardman, L. E. Kazis, S. E. Martin, R. A. Horney, A. L. Wiseman, D. S. Kernodle, R. P. Smith, A. L. Baltch, C. Handanos, B. Catto, L. Montalvo, M. Everson, W. Blackburn, M. Thakore, S. T. Brown, L. Lutwick, D. Norwood, J. Bernstein, C. Bacheller, B. Ribner, L. W. P. Church, K. H. Wilson, P. Guduru, R. Cooper, J. Lentino, R. J. Hamill, A. B. Gorin, V. Gordan, D. Wagner, C. Robinson, P. DeJace, R. Greenfield, L. Beck, M. Bittner, H. R. Schumacher, F. Silverblatt, J. Schmitt, E. Wong, M. A. K. Ryan, J. Figueroa, C. Nice, J. R. Feussner, and V. A. C. Group. 2004. Benefits and harms of doxycycline treatment for Gulf War veterans' illnesses: A randomized, double-blind, placebo-controlled trial. *Annals of Internal Medicine* 141(2):85-94.

Escobar, J. I., M. A. Gara, A. M. Diaz-Martinez, A. Interian, M. Warman, L. A. Allen, R. L. Woolfolk, E. Jahn, and D. Rodgers. 2007. Effectiveness of a time-limited cognitive behavior therapy type intervention among primary care patients with medically unexplained symptoms. *Annals of Family Medicine* 5(4):328-335.

Guarino, P., P. Peduzzi, S. T. Donta, C. C. Engel, D. J. Clauw, D. A. Williams, J. S. Skinner, A. Barkhuizen, L. E. Kazis, and J. R. Feussner. 2001. A multicenter two by two factorial trial of cognitive behavioral therapy and aerobic exercise for Gulf War veterans' illnesses: Design of a Veterans Affairs cooperative study (CSP #470). *Controlled Clinical Trials* 22(3):310-332.

Lidbeck, J. 2003. Group therapy for somatization disorders in primary care: Maintenance of treatment goals of short cognitive-behavioural treatment one-and-a-half-year follow-up. *Acta Psychiatrica Scandinavica* 107(6):449-456.

Lincoln, A. E., D. A. Helmer, A. I. Schneiderman, M. Li, H. Copeland, M. K. Prisco, M. T. Wallin, H. K. Kang, and B. H. Natelson. 2006. The War-Related Illness and Injury Study Centers: A resource for deployment-related health concerns. *Military Medicine* 171(7):577-585.

Martin, A., E. Rauh, M. Fichter, and W. Rief. 2007. A one-session treatment for patients suffering from medically unexplained symptoms in primary care: A randomized clinical trial. *Psychosomatics* 48(4):294-303.

Mori, D. L., S. Sogg, P. Guarino, J. Skinner, D. Williams, A. Barkhuizen, C. Engel, D. Clauw, S. Donta, and P. Peduzzi. 2006. Predictors of exercise compliance in individuals with Gulf War veterans illnesses: Department of Veterans Affairs cooperative study 470. *Military Medicine* 171(9):917-923.

Muller, T., M. Mannel, H. Murck, and V. W. Rahlfs. 2004. Treatment of somatoform disorders with St. John's wort: A randomized, double-blind and placebo-controlled trial. *Psychosomatic Medicine* 66(4):538-547.

Peters, S., I. Stanley, M. Rose, S. Kaney, and P. Salmon. 2002. A randomized controlled trial of group aerobic exercise in primary care patients with persistent, unexplained physical symptoms. *Family Practice* 19(6):665-674.

Reinhard, M. J. 2012. *Complementary and Alternative Medicine (CAM) and Chronic Multi-Symptom Illness*. Presentation at the Second Committee Meeting, February 29, 2012, Washington, DC.

Reisinger, H. S., S. C. Hunt, A. L. Burgo-Black, and M. A. Agarwal. 2012. A population approach to mitigating the long-term health effects of combat deployments. *Preventing Chronic Disease* 9:E54.

Rief, W., G. Bleichhardt, and B. Timmer. 2002. Group therapy for somatoform disorders: Treatment guidelines, acceptance, and process quality. *Verhaltenstherapie* 12(3):183-191.

Sharpe, M., J. Walker, C. Williams, J. Stone, J. Cavanagh, G. Murray, I. Butcher, R. Duncan, S. Smith, and A. Carson. 2011. Guided self-help for functional (psychogenic) symptoms a randomized controlled efficacy trial. *Neurology* 77(6):564-572.

Sumathipala, A., S. Hewege, R. Hanwella, and A. H. Mann. 2000. Randomized controlled trial of cognitive behaviour therapy for repeated consultations for medically unexplained complaints: A feasibility study in Sri Lanka. *Psychological Medicine* 30(4):747-757.

Sumathipala, A., S. Siribaddana, M. Abeysingha, P. De Silva, M. Dewey, M. Prince, and A. Mann. 2008. Cognitive-behavioural therapy v. structured care for medically unexplained symptoms: Randomised controlled trial. *British Journal of Psychiatry* 193(1):51-59.

VA (Department of Veterans Affairs). 2011. *VA Centers of Excellence in Primary Care Education*. http://www.va.gov/oaa/rfp_coe.asp (accessed September 19, 2012).

VA and DOD (Department of Defense). 2001a. *Clinical Practice Guideline for Post-Deployment Health Evaluation and Management, Version 1.2.*

VA and DOD. 2001b. *Clinical Practice Guideline for the Management of Medically Unexplained Symptoms: Chronic Pain and Fatigue.* http://www.healthquality.va.gov/mus/mus_fulltext.pdf (accessed September 19, 2012).

VA and DOD. 2009a. *Clinical Practice Guideline for the Management of Substance Use Disorders (SUD).* http://www.healthquality.va.gov/sud/sud_full_601f.pdf (accessed September 19, 2012).

VA and DOD. 2009b. *Clinical Practice Guideline: Management of Concussion/Mild Traumatic Brain Injury.* http://www.healthquality.va.gov/mtbi/concussion_mtbi_full_1_0.pdf (accessed September 19, 2012).

VA and DOD. 2009c. *Clinical Practice Guideline: Management of Major Depressive Disorder (MDD).* http://www.healthquality.va.gov/MDD_FULL_3c.pdf (accessed September 19, 2012).

VA and DOD. 2010a. *Clinical Practice Guideline for Management of Post-Traumatic Stress.* http://www.healthquality.va.gov/ptsd/PTSD-FULL-2010a.pdf (accessed September 19, 2012).

VA and DOD. 2010b. *Clinical Practice Guideline: Management of Opioid Therapy for Chronic Pain.* http://www.healthquality.va.gov/COT_312_Full-er.pdf (accessed September 19, 2012).

Volz, H. P., H. Murck, S. Kasper, and H. J. Moller. 2002. St. John's wort extract (Li 160) in somatoform disorders: Results of a placebo-controlled trial. *Psychopharmacology* 164(3):294-300.

Zaby, A., J. Heider, and A. Schroder. 2008. Waiting, relaxation, or cognitive-behavioral therapy: How effective is outpatient group therapy for somatoform symptoms? *Zeitschrift für Klinische Psychologie und Psychotherapie* 37(1):15-23.

Appendix A

Committee Biographic Sketches

Bernard M. Rosof, MD, MACP (*Chair*), is chairman of the Board of Directors of Huntington Hospital, which is part of the North Shore–LIJ Health System. He has been affiliated with Huntington Hospital since 1963 and has held a number of administrative positions. Dr. Rosof is also chief executive officer of the Quality in Health Care Advisory Group, LLC, and is a professor of medicine at Hofstra North Shore–LIJ School of Medicine. He is recognized for his work on issues of health quality, patient safety, clinical practice guidelines, and performance improvement. Dr. Rosof practiced internal medicine and gastroenterology for 29 years. He has served on several Institute of Medicine committees, including serving as chair of the Committee on Identifying Effective Treatments for Gulf War Veterans' Health Problems. Dr. Rosof is a member of the Board of Directors of the National Quality Forum and has chaired committees and task forces for the State of New York, the American Medical Association, and various specialty societies. He is a master of the American College of Physicians and chair emeritus of the college's Board of Regents. Dr. Rosof received his medical degree from the New York University School of Medicine and completed a fellowship in gastroenterology at the Yale University School of Medicine.

Diana D. Cardenas, MD, MHA, is professor and chair of the Department of Rehabilitation Medicine of the University of Miami (UM) Leonard M. Miller School of Medicine. She is also the principal investigator of the South Florida Spinal Cord Injury Model System, an R&D project funded by the National Institute on Disability and Rehabilitation Research, in

195

which her current research focus is musculoskeletal pain. She is also program director of the UM/Jackson Memorial Hospital Spinal Cord Injury Medicine Fellowship and chief of service of rehabilitation medicine at Jackson Memorial Hospital in Miami, Florida. She has served as chair of the Research Advisory and Advocacy Committee of the American Academy of Physical Medicine and Rehabilitation (1997–2000), a member of the Board of Directors of the American Spinal Injury Association, and chair of the National Institutes of Health National Advisory Board on Medical Rehabilitation Research (2007–2008). She has published more than 200 articles, chapters, abstracts, and books on epidemiology, clinical trials, and outcomes research related to the secondary conditions and medical complications associated with a number of disabilities, including spinal-cord injury, traumatic brain injury, chronic neuropathic pain, and nociceptive pain. In 2004, she was elected to the Institute of Medicine (IOM). She has served on three prior IOM committees (the Committee on Assessing Rehabilitation Science and Engineering, the Committee on Injury Prevention and Control, and the Committee on Improving the Disability Decision Process). She served on the IOM Board on Military and Veterans Health from 2006 to 2009 and for 1 more year when it became the Board on the Health of Select Populations. She maintains a clinical practice in addition to her administrative and research activities.

Frank V. deGruy III, MD, is Woodward-Chisholm Professor and chair of the Department of Family Medicine of the University of Colorado School of Medicine. Dr. deGruy has also held academic appointments in the Departments of Family Medicine of Case Western Reserve University, Duke University, and the College of Medicine at the University of South Alabama. He served as chair of the National Advisory Committee for the Robert Wood Johnson Foundation's Depression in Primary Care program. Dr. deGruy is past president of the Collaborative Family Healthcare Association, is chair of the Board of Directors of the Family Physicians Inquiries Network, and is the president of the North American Primary Care Research Group. He is the author of more than 100 papers, chapters, books, editorials, and reviews and has been the principal investigator on a number of research and training grants having to do with somatization, mental disorders in primary care, and primary care practice redesign. Dr. deGruy received his MD from the College of Medicine at the University of South Alabama.

Douglas A. Drossman, MD, is adjunct professor of medicine and psychiatry at the University of North Carolina (UNC) and former codirector of the UNC Center for Functional GI & Motility Disorders in the Division of Gastroenterology and Hepatology. He has a longstanding interest in the evaluation of care for gastrointestinal (GI) disorders that are difficult to diagnose and treat. He began a program of research in functional GI disorders 30 years ago and has received numerous National Institutes of Health (NIH) grants in that field. He has published more than 500 books, articles, and abstracts related to the epidemiology, psychosocial, and quality-of-life assessment, design of treatment trials, and outcomes of research in GI disorders, and he was associate editor of the journal *Gastroenterology* and gastroenterology editor of the *Merck Manual*. He has served on two previous Institute of Medicine *Gulf War and Health* committees—the ones that produced *Physiologic, Psychologic, and Psychosocial Effects of Deployment-Related Stress* and *Health Effects of Serving in the Gulf War, Update 2009*. Dr. Drossman is president of the Rome Foundation, an international organization that sets guidelines and standards for diagnosis and care of patients who have functional GI disorders, and is president of the Drossman Center for Education and Practice of Biopsychosocial Care, which develops training programs for physicians to learn communication skills to improve the patient–provider relationship. Dr. Drossman received his MD from the Albert Einstein College of Medicine and fellowships in psychosomatic medicine at the University of Rochester and in gastroenterology at UNC.

Francesca C. Dwamena, MD, MS, is professor and acting chair of the Department of Medicine of Michigan State University. Dr. Dwamena also is an adjunct professor of psychiatry and an attending physician for the Michigan State University Health Team and at Sparrow Hospital. She specializes in psychosocial medicine and is coauthor of a major text on medical interviewing. Dr. Dwamena has more than 40 published works on many aspects of clinical and primary medicine, including the identification of and treatment for medically unexplained symptoms. She received her MD from Howard University College of Medicine and her MS in epidemiology and a certificate in psychosocial medicine from Michigan State University.

Javier I. Escobar, MD, MSc, is associate dean for global health and professor of psychiatry and family medicine at the University of Medicine and Dentistry of New Jersey–Robert Wood Johnson Medical School. He has been an active researcher in clinical psychopharmacology, psychiatry, psychiatric epidemiology, psychiatric diagnosis, cross-cultural medicine, mental disorders in primary care, and treatment of somatoform disorders. Dr. Escobar has been the principal investigator of several National Institutes of Health–funded grants in medically unexplained symptoms, mentoring of young researchers, and mental health–primary-care collaborations. He has published more than 200 scientific articles in books and journals and has served on a number of advisory committees and task forces, including those for the National Institute of Mental Health, the World Health Organization, the Food and Drug Administration, the Department of Veterans Affairs, and the Robert Wood Johnson Foundation. Dr. Escobar received his MD from Universidad de Antioquia, Medellin, Colombia, and did his specialty training and obtained a master's degree in psychiatry–medical genetics at the University of Minnesota.

Wayne A. Gordon, PhD, is Jack Nash Professor of Rehabilitation Medicine and vice chair of the Department of Rehabilitation Medicine at the Mount Sinai School of Medicine. He is a neuropsychologist and the director of the Mount Sinai Brain Injury Research Center. Dr. Gordon's recent research has focused on cognitive rehabilitation and other types of behavioral interventions to improve the functioning of people who have traumatic brain injury (TBI) and on the secondary conditions that are associated with TBI. In 2009, he received the Robert L. Moody Prize for Distinguished Initiatives in Brain Injury Research and Rehabilitation. In 2010, he received the Caveness Award from the Brain Injury Association of America, and in 2011 he received the Gold Key Award from the American Congress of Rehabilitation Medicine. He is a member of the Board of the Ontario Neurotrauma Foundation and the Brain Injury Association of America. He is past president of the American Congress of Rehabilitation Medicine. Dr. Gordon has published more than 125 articles and book chapters and has presented nationally and internationally on his research. He has served on peer-review panels for the National Institutes of Health, the Centers for Disease Control and Prevention, the National Institute on Disability and Rehabilitation Research, the Department of Defense, and the Department of Veterans Affairs. He served on the Institute of Medicine Committee on Traumatic Brain Injury. Dr. Gordon received his PhD from Yeshiva University.

Isabel V. Hoverman, MD, MACP, is an internist in private practice in Austin, Texas, with 35 years of experience. She is also an assistant professor at the University of Texas Medical Branch at Galveston. Her career began at the Houston VA Medical Center. She has served in several leadership positions for professional organizations and has been active in quality and safety in health care at the local and national levels. She was on two previous Institute of Medicine (IOM) *Gulf War and Health* committees—the ones that produced *Identifying Effective Treatments for Gulf War Veterans' Health Problems* and *Measuring the Health of Gulf War Veterans*. She has also served on three other IOM committees: the Committee on a National Center on War-Related Illness and Post-Deployment Health Issues, the Committee on the Evaluation of the Department of Veterans Affairs Uniform Case Assessment Protocol, and the Committee to Evaluate the Medicare Peer Review Organization Program Evaluation Plan. Dr. Hoverman received her MD from the Duke University Medical School.

Wayne Jonas, MD, DHT, FAAFP, is Samueli Institute's president and chief executive officer. He has had a long and distinguished career as a student, practitioner, and researcher of conventional medicine and complementary and alternative medical (CAM) practices. His experience includes service as an administrator, an international conference chairman, a speaker, a panel moderator, a peer reviewer, and an author of books and scientific articles on conventional and CAM topics. He is currently associate professor of family medicine at the Uniformed Services University of the Health Sciences and professor of family medicine at Georgetown University School of Medicine. Dr. Jonas served as the director of the Office of Alternative Medicine at the National Institutes of Health from 1995 to 1999; before that, he was the director of the Medical Research Fellowship of the Walter Reed Army Institute of Research. He served for 24 years as an Army medical officer. At Samueli Institute, he has led the development of major whole-systems evaluation programs, including Optimal Healing Environments, Total Force Fitness, and the Wellness Initiative for the Nation. His current research interests include the placebo effect, cancer, the biologic effects of low-level toxin exposures, homeopathy, spiritual healing, and the quality of research methods on outcomes. Dr. Jonas received his MD from the Wake Forest University School of Medicine.

Joanna G. Katzman, MD, MSPH, is director of the University of New Mexico (UNM) School of Medicine Pain Center and the Project ECHO tele-ECHO Chronic Pain and Headache Clinic. She is an associate professor in neurology at the University of New Mexico School of Medicine and is the deputy chief medical officer for clinical integration and ambulatory services for the UNM Health System. The UNM School of Medicine Pain Center was awarded the 2011 American Pain Society Clinical Center of Excellence. Dr. Katzman is helping the Department of Veterans Affairs and Department of Defense in replication of ECHO throughout military patient care centers. Dr. Katzman received her MD from Yale University School of Medicine. She completed her neurology residency and fellowship training in neurorehabilitation at the University of California, Los Angeles, Medical Center. She also holds an MS in public health.

Elaine L. Larson, RN, PhD, FAAN, CIC, is associate dean for research and a professor of pharmaceutical and therapeutic research at the Columbia University School of Nursing and a professor of epidemiology at Columbia University Mailman School of Public Health. She is a former dean of Georgetown University School of Nursing. Dr. Larson has been a member of the Board of Directors of the National Foundation for Infectious Diseases. She is a member of the Institute of Medicine and has participated in numerous activities of the National Academies. She has been an editor of the *American Journal of Infection Control* since 1994 and has published more than 200 journal articles, 4 books, and a number of book chapters in infection prevention, epidemiology, and clinical research. Dr. Larson received her MA and PhD from the University of Washington.

Stephen Ray Mitchell, MD, is the Joseph Butenas Professor and dean of medical education at Georgetown University and has been a member of the Georgetown University Hospital faculty since 1988, also serving as program director in internal medicine and starting an innovative pediatrics residency program in conjunction with Pew Charitable Trusts and the Partnerships in Quality Education. He is an expert in the field of adult and pediatric rheumatology and is a founding Fellow of the American College of Rheumatology. In 2004, Dr. Mitchell was inducted into mastership of the American College of Physicians—the highest honor of the college, bestowed on only 600 living members of the 150,000-member organization—and he serves on the Council of Deans of the Association of American Medical Colleges. A veteran, he completed 8 years on active duty, including temporary service in the Persian Gulf with the 82nd Airborne Division before the Gulf War. He received his MD from the University of North Carolina and trained in internal medicine and pediatrics at North Carolina Memorial Hospital and completed a fellowship in rheumatology at Georgetown University and the District of Columbia VA Medical Center.

Karen A. Robinson, PhD, MSc, is an assistant professor of medicine, epidemiology, and health policy and management and a codirector of the Evidence-Based Practice Center of Johns Hopkins University. Her work has focused on evidence-based health care and health informatics. Dr. Robinson is experienced in conducting systematic reviews to assess the efficacy and effectiveness of therapies. She has led and participated in many activities supporting the Cochrane Collaboration, including being an editor for two Cochrane review groups. Dr. Robinson received her MSc in health sciences from the University of Waterloo, Ontario, and her PhD in epidemiology from the Johns Hopkins University Bloomberg School of Public Health.

Kasisomayajula (Vish) Viswanath, PhD, is an associate professor in the Department of Society, Human Development, and Health at the Harvard School of Public Health; a faculty member in the Center for Community-Based Research at the Dana-Farber Cancer Institute; and director of the Health Communication Core of the Dana-Farber/Harvard Cancer Center. Dr. Viswanath's current research focuses on documenting the link between inequalities in communication and health disparities and on addressing the disparities through communication and dissemination. He is equally concerned with bridging the gap between "discovery" and "delivery" and is working toward translating knowledge to influence public-health policy and practice. Dr. Viswanath was appointed chair of the Board of Scientific Counselors of the National Center for Health Marketing of the Centers for Disease Control and Prevention. Before his current position at Harvard, Dr. Viswanath was the acting associate director of the Behavioral Research Program in the Division of Cancer Control and Populations Sciences and a senior scientist in the Health Communication and Informatics Research Branch of the National Cancer Institute; on the faculty of the Ohio State University School of Journalism and Communication with an adjunct appointment in the School of Public Health; and a center scholar with Ohio State University's Center for Health Outcomes, Policy, and Evaluation Studies. Dr. Viswanath is active in many professional organizations. He has published extensively on a variety of topics spanning health communication, social epidemiology, and social and health behavior in both health and communication journals. Dr. Viswanath received his PhD from the University of Minnesota.

Lori Zoellner, PhD, is an associate professor in the Department of Psychology of the University of Washington. She is director of the University of Washington's Center for Anxiety and Traumatic Stress. Her research focuses on understanding biopsychosocial mechanisms that underlie the prevention of and treatment for posttraumatic stress disorder. She received her PhD in clinical psychology with a minor in behavioral neuroscience from the University of California, Los Angeles.

Appendix B

Possible Factors Underlying Chronic Multisymptom Illness

Chronic multisymptom illness (CMI)—like several other syndromes, including fibromyalgia, chronic fatigue syndrome (CFS), and irritable bowel syndrome (IBS)—lacks characteristic biomarkers. In the absence of other diseases that would explain the symptoms, its diagnosis is based on symptom criteria. CMI can consist of diverse symptoms that vary among people or even within the same person over time. The symptoms may be related to central nervous system upregulation (amplification) of neural signals that have a somatic or visceral origin rather than originating exclusively in bodily conditions. That mechanism is similar to the current understanding of IBS in deployed Gulf War veterans, which appears to develop by the combination of gastroenteritis, leading to gut mucosal immune dysfunction and inflammation, and impairment of the brain's ability to reduce or down-regulate neural signals from the gastrointestinal tract related to the deployment experience (Drossman, 1999; IOM, 2010; Spiller and Garsed, 2009). The dysregulation of the "brain–gut axis," malfunctioning of the visceral signaling regulatory system, leads to the characteristic symptoms of IBS.

Although the degree to which the brain enhances neurologic signals from the body in CMI has yet to be determined, it is recognized that the brain's ability to filter incoming signals is highly modifiable by environmental and psychologic factors. For example, the number of symptoms that people report correlates with psychologic and environmental factors, including levels of anxiety and depression and the degree of stress after exposure to abuse or war trauma (Bair, 2003; IOM, 2008; Vaccarino et al., 2009; Zaubler and Katon, 1996). Such correlations do not imply that the symptoms reported are indicative of a psychiatric disorder. In those who have pain, these correlations are explained in part by the effects of stressors on limbic areas of the brain (in particular, the cingulate cortex) that are associated with pain regulation. For example, a history of physical and sexual abuse is associated with increased reports of pain in people who have IBS, and increased pain correlates with enhanced activation of the midcingulate cortex, an area at the interface of pain regulation and emotional input (Ringel et al., 2008). In addition, peripheral inflammatory states associated with increased cytokine activation may in turn alter brain functioning, producing "sickness behavior." These phenomena may help to explain the emotional distress and increased symptom awareness associated with CMI (Dantzer et al., 2008). That putative mechanism is illustrated in Figure B-1, which demonstrates that somatic and visceral sensations (for example, muscle pain, fatigue, and abdominal pain) are experienced as symptoms only when the signal amplitude is above the brain's perception threshold. Thus, peripheral neural signals arising from an injury might be above the perception threshold and be experienced as a symptom, and other regulatory signals (for example, increased gut signals after eating) might be received in the brain but not experienced as a symptom unless one overeats or has a gastrointestinal disorder, such as functional dyspepsia. In addition, the brain's ability to downregulate incoming signals (that is, to raise the threshold level) will depend on regulatory processes and the person's cognitive and emotional state. Thus, injuring oneself might not be experienced as a symptom when one is distracted during a sports event until the event is

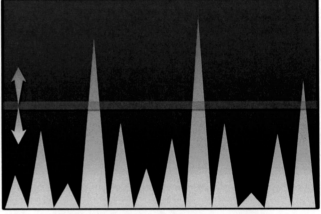

FIGURE B-1 Putative mechanism by which the body perceives symptoms.

over. Conversely, anxiety about an injury and hypervigilance to the affected part can lead to increased pain. In CMI, central factors may lead to a lower sensation threshold and, if this is the case, centrally targeted treatments would probably have therapeutic value by increasing sensation thresholds, as occurs in treatment for other conditions, such as fibromyalgia, CFS, and IBS. There is some evidence that patients who have similar somatic symptoms have higher concentrations of substance P (which transmits pain) in their blood and cerebrospinal fluid than people who do not have such symptoms (Clauw, 2009). In those patients, direct pressure on the skin or inflation of a balloon in the esophagus causes pain at a much lower level of pressure than in people who do not have these somatic symptoms.

In addition, central measures of hormonal stress, such as an altered response of the hypothalamic-pituitary-adrenal axis, reveal an inappropriate flattened response to additional stress that may reflect a more sustained central overactivity in patients who have visceral hypersensitivity (such as IBS) or somatic hypersensitivity (such as fibromyalgia) (Clauw, 2009).

Nonrestorative sleep can be reproduced in normal volunteers who are subjected to disruption of deep stage four sleep and is a typical sleep pattern in patients who have IBS. When deep stage four sleep is repeatedly disrupted, affected people can develop myalgia, heightened pain, presence of tender points on examination, and disrupted sleep patterns afterward. Further research is needed to assess whether use of programs and agents that restore a better sleep pattern may also lead to improvement in other symptoms.

In summary, the multiple symptoms of CMI, like the symptoms associated with other functional somatic syndromes, may arise from at least two factors: an impairment of the brain in its downregulating of incoming nerve signals originating in the body and an increase in or amplification of bodily nerve signals for any of a variety of reasons (such as injury or infection). The degree to which those factors interact in CMI is an important topic for future research.

REFERENCES

Bair, M. J. 2003. Depression and pain mortality: A literature review. *Archives of Internal Medicine* 163(20):2433-2445.

Clauw, D. J. 2009. Fibromyalgia: An overview. *American Journal of Medicine* 122(12 Suppl.):S3-S13.

Dantzer, R., J. C. O'Connor, G. G. Freund, R. W. Johnson, and K. W. Kelley. 2008. From inflammation to sickness and depression: When the immune system subjugates the brain. *Nature Reviews Neuroscience* 9(1):46-56.

Drossman, D. A. 1999. Mind over matter in the postinfective irritable bowel. *Gut* 44(3):306-307.

IOM (Institute of Medicine). 2008. *Gulf War and Health, Volume 6: Physiologic, Psychologic, and Psychosocial Effects of Deployment-related Stress.* Washington, DC: The National Academies Press.

IOM. 2010. *Gulf War and Health, Volume 8: Update of Health Effects of Serving in the Gulf War*. Washington, DC: The National Academies Press.

Ringel, Y., D. A. Drossman, J. L. Leserman, B. Y. Suyenobu, K. Wilber, and W. Lin. 2008. Effect of abuse history on pain reports and brain responses to aversive visceral stimulation: An FMRI study. *Gastroenterology* 134(2):396-404.

Spiller, R., and K. Garsed. 2009. Postinfectious irritable bowel syndrome. *Gastroenterology* 136(6):1979-1988.

Vaccarino, A. L., T. L. Stills, K. R. Evans, and A. H. Kalali. 2009. Multiple pain complaints in patients with major depressive disorder. *Psychosomatic Medicine* 71(2):159-162.

Zaubler, T. S., and W. J. Katon. 1996. Panic disorder and medical comorbidity: A review of the medical and psychiatric literature. *Bulletin of the Menninger Clinic* 20(2 Suppl. A):A12-A38.

Appendix C

Examples of Effective and Ineffective Patient–Clinician Discussions

As noted in Chapter 6, the foundation of a treatment plan for a veteran who has chronic multisymptom illness is the establishment of an effective patient–clinician relationship. The basis of an effective relationship is proper interview technique. To assist with clinician training to improve interviewing skills, the Department of Veterans Affairs may want to consider developing videos based on the illustrative scripts in Boxes C-1 and C-2 that demonstrate ineffective and effective patient–patient discussions.

There are several observations to address in the conversation in Box C-1. First, there was no eye contact when the doctor greeted the patient; the doctor was reviewing the chart. The flow of the discussion was not effective in gathering information, because the doctor asked closed-ended, multiple-choice questions and interrupted the patient twice while the patient was attempting to say something. There was no opportunity for the patient to tell the story, and the communication was passive. In addition, toward the end of the conversation it was difficult to follow the flow of the conversation because the doctor and patient were working from different agendas. Then the doctor seemed to close the discussion by offering to order tests, perhaps in an effort to reassure the patient. When the patient raised concern about the diagnosis and whether it was Gulf War syndrome, the doctor did not address this concern. Furthermore, the doctor disregarded the validity of the diagnosis, focusing more on seeing that the tests would be done to exclude other conditions as a means of reassuring the patient. Finally, the doctor indicated an interest in placing the patient on an antidepressant if the tests were negative but gave no explanation as

---

BOX C-1
Example of an *Ineffective* Patient–Clinician Discussion

Doctor. "How can I help you?" (looking at chart)

Patient. "I developed another flareup of whatever I have . . . the fatigue, muscle aches, stomach pain, and terrible nausea, when I came back from vacation . . . (pause) . . . (pensive) I . . ."

Dr. "Was this like what you had before?" (interrupting)

Pt. "Yes . . . well, almost . . . I think."

Dr. "Was it made worse by food?" (looks up)

Pt. "Yes, I think so."

Dr. "Did you have fever? or chest pain?" (leaning forward)

Pt. "Well, yes, I think, . . . but I didn't take my temperature" (looks down)

Dr. "So you had fever and chest pain?"

Pt. "Uh no, well, the pain wasn't bad . . . I guess. . . . Dr., I'm really worried about this."

Dr. "Let me go ahead and schedule you for some blood work and maybe another X-ray. It'll probably be ok, but this way we'll be sure there is nothing to worry about."

Pt. "But what do I have? I saw on the veterans website that some other people had the same things, and they called it Gulf War syndrome. Is that what I have?"

Dr. "Most people aren't sure whether that's a real medical condition, so I want to rule out anything else that we can treat. If the studies are negative, I'd like to put you on an antidepressant to make you feel more comfortable."

Pt. (looking confused) "I'm not depressed. . . . I just can't deal with the pain and nausea. I . . ."

Dr. (interrupting) "I didn't say you were depressed. It can help the symptoms. Let's see what the tests show."

---

to why. The doctor's comment led the patient to infer that the medicine was being used for depression, which he did not think he had.

It is noteworthy that although the number of verbal exchanges is the same in both conversations, the content and the messages communicated are richer in the second one (Box C-2), with far more clinical content and probably greater effectiveness in building the patient–clinician relationship. It is clear that the doctor is fully engaged in helping the patient. The doctor listens actively, gives the patient the opportunity to tell his story, and responds to the patient's comments and concerns. Validating statements are used (for example, "I can see how much this is really affecting your

BOX C-2
Example of an *Effective* Patient–Clinician Discussion

Doctor. "How can I help you?" (concerned, looking at patient)

Patient. "I developed another flareup of whatever I have . . . the muscle aches, stomach pain, and terrible nausea, when I came back from vacation . . . (pause) . . . (pensive) I . . ."

Dr. "Yes?"

Pt. "I was about to start my new position as floor supervisor, and . . . and then all this happened."

Dr. "Oh, I see . . ." (pause)

Pt. "(Continues) I started getting those muscle aches and that fatigue, then the cramps came on right here (points to lower abdomen), and it got worse after eating. It felt like the flu. I felt warm but didn't take my temperature. So I knew it was getting worse again, so I came in to see you. I'm really getting worried about this."

Dr. "Hmmm . . . how so?"

Pt. "Well, it's really starting to cut into things. I'm afraid to do any sports or go out to eat, and I'm worried about my job. I'm irritable and don't think I'm doing a good job at home. But my wife is really terrific. Then you know I got this promotion, but what am I going to do if I can't do the job because of this?"

Dr. "I can see how much this is really affecting your life."

Pt. "That's right; sometimes I don't think anyone understands. Doctor, what do I have? I've been reading this veterans website, and some of the people have the same problems. They're calling it Gulf War syndrome."

Dr. "Yes, it's gotta be hard when it seems that no one really understands what you're going through. You know, there is a lot of discussion about Gulf War syndrome, or what we now call chronic multisymptom illness, or CMI. You are not alone with this, and medical researchers and the VA medical system are working to understand the causes and find treatments. I can see from your records that you have had a full medical evaluation on a couple of occasions, and since the symptoms haven't changed I believe you do have CMI. So I'd really like for us to focus more on ways to manage your symptoms."

Pt. "That sounds good, so what do you want to do?"

Dr. "Well, the first thing is that I want to work together with you on this. There is no magic pill, but I have several ideas that we can discuss that may help you get back to the life you want. I can see that these symptoms are so bad that they also affect your emotional well-being, your family relationships, and your quality of life. So, while we are

continued

BOX C-2 Continued

working on getting some relief for the symptoms, I want you to also see a colleague of mine, a psychologist who will work with you to develop coping strategies and help you find ways get back to a more normal lifestyle. I also would like you to put you on a certain type of antidepressants that can help reduce some of the pain and discomfort you are experiencing. They act on nerve pathways from the brain to your body to help block pain signals, and they often can be used in lower dosages than are used for depression."

Pt. "So, it's not because I'm depressed?"

Dr. "Well, medicines have different effects. Aspirin can relieve pain and also prevent a heart attack. Certain antidepressants are also used to treat a variety of painful conditions like body pain, irritable bowel, and even pain from diabetes. Also, if all of this is making you feel depressed, it can help for that as well."

Pt. "Okay. I'll give it a try. Thank you, doctor."

Alternative ending:

Dr. "Well, the first thing is that I want to continue to work with you on this. There is no magic pill, but I have several ideas to help reduce the symptoms and work to get you back to the life you want. There is a VA program that is designed to provide a team approach to the treatment that addresses not only your physical symptoms but also your emotional well-being and your quality of life. I'd like you to sign up with that program, and then you would come back to see me in 3–4 weeks to go over your progress. How does that sound?"

Pt. "That sounds great. Thanks so much for your help."

life"), and the patient is informed that he is not alone in his experience. This allows the patient to say more about how the illness is affecting his life and about the stress of getting a promotion while being uncertain about how well he can do the work. Then the doctor validates the illness, and the conversation moves toward working collaboratively with the patient on the treatment. Finally, the recommendation for the psychologist and antidepressant (or the VA program) is addressed in a fashion that will be understandable and relevant to the patient's interests and needs.

Index